Nobody Walks Alone

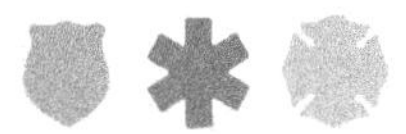

Overcoming the Darkness of EMS

Dale M. Bayliss

Nobody Walks Alone

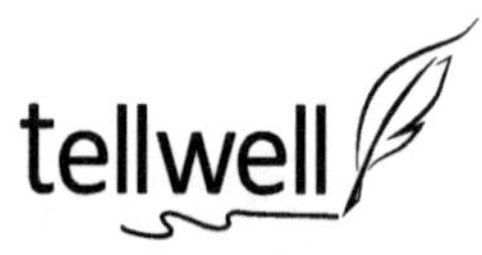

Tellwell Talent
www.tellwell.ca

ISBN
978-0-2288-0598-4 (Hardcover)
978-0-2288-0597-7 (Paperback)
978-0-2288-0599-1 (eBook)

Let your desire to help people be one thing that no one can ever take away from you. You can help as many people as time allows. You can achieve any level of care provider possible. Go as far as you need to go to make a difference. Only time and perseverance will reveal the surest and safest paths to be successful in life.

—Dale M. Bayliss

Dedication

This book is dedicated to the many EMS, nursing, medical and allied health students whom I have had the privilege to educate or mentor. My success stories and our tragedies are shared with my many co-workers as well as my mentors. There have been many people who have positively influenced me, making No One Walks Alone – Overcoming the Darkness of EMS *possible. For that I'm truly grateful.*

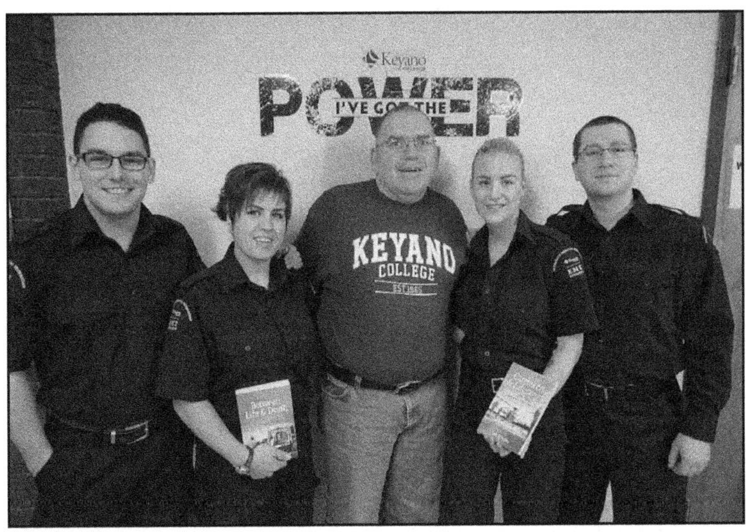

This book is my chance to inspire the people around me, especially within the EMS industry, in a positive way. If nothing else, I hope to show you all that there can be great outcomes, despite the trials and tribulations we all face. By following our dreams of making this world a better place, we can change the world around us. I have learned so much from the many great people whom I've had the privilege to work alongside over my lifetime. Hanging out with great people influences one's life and gives one hope during difficult days and

nights. My hope is that the people who come after me will carry on this legacy of caring and compassion, and of making a difference in the lives of others. My only request is that they carry the passion to help others forward.

We need to show up as a team and leave as a team, while always working as one. Teamwork increases the chance of better outcomes for the lives we hold in our hands. It's vital that you know that you, too, can make a difference and influence the outcome if you simply try your best in your role. During my career, I always tried to do my best, no matter the situation, in order to create a legacy that will be carried on for all the right reasons.

Please remember that everyone matters.
Every one of you.

"Sometimes we need to bend the rules to save
a life, but we must not break our moral code, destroy
our ethics or lose our soul along the way."

—Dale M. Bayliss

Table of Contents

Preface

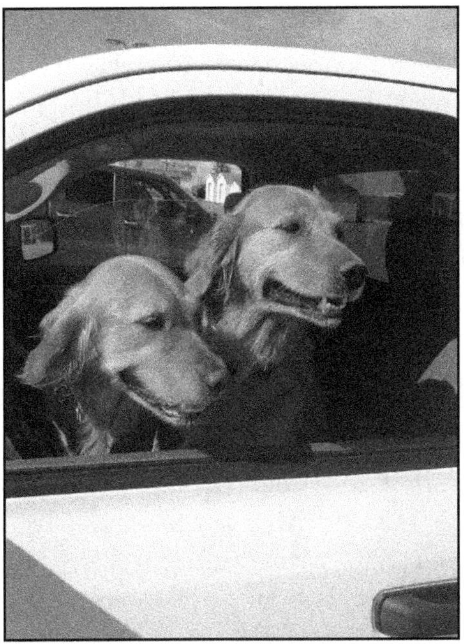

Pebbles and Tinsel – my 24/7 backup

My reason for being is very simple. I figured out at a young age that I wanted to help people. Truthfully, I *needed* to help people. It's what I was meant to do. Helping people gave my life a purpose. It has taken me a lifetime of learning and growing to develop into the person I am today. Emergency Medical Services (EMS) was my chosen pathway in life, and it took ten years from the day I began working toward it to finally become a paramedic, but it was worth every second.

My dual careers as a registered nurse and an advanced care paramedic evolved over time. I was very dedicated to achieving both goals, and often worked on them both at the same time. From a very young age I knew I would become a paramedic but achieving that goal was not easy. As with anything that requires a higher level of education and training, the EMS field requires dedication and commitment to be successful. Working as a registered nurse is a very rewarding occupation, but it is a completely different occupation than working as a paramedic, even though some challenges are similar. I could have become a farmer, a welder, a builder or a truck driver but none of these were my calling in life. I felt destined to be a teacher, a mentor, helping people and directly or indirectly saving lives. At the end of the day, my roles define me as a person and as a professional. After every shift I would come home, and my golden retrievers would be there to help me cope with the effect of bad calls. They were part of the EMS team even if people never saw them. They were always on my team.

Throughout my life, I've had many close calls. I have been physically hurt several times. I've gotten a few grey hairs, as well as some cool scars to show for it. It was not only my safety that I was worried about, but also the safety of my partners and co-workers when we responded to our calls. We were often in charge of the well-being or safety of other people around us, as well, such as the families of victims or bystanders. I was not immune to being hurt, but due to my size, strength and determination I was tougher than most. It's not always about size and strength, though; it's about the determination to succeed and to overcome the hurdles we all face from time to time. I have bleed for others, I have been left hurt and scared, but I got back up.

When we are young we don't appreciate the size and complexity of our world. The older I got, the smaller the world seemed to get, and living or working within different sets of rules and organizations became more complex. The ability to adapt to a constantly changing world is a requirement to be able to function and stay safe. Some days the rules, or the organizational structure, can break you down. If you let your guard down and let the negative in, it can overpower your optimism. As Granny Bayliss would often say, "If you can't say something nice then don't say anything." She also warned us all that "if you drive like hell, that's where you will end up" and both quotes were pretty good advice. The best way to stay out of hell is to avoid that general direction. The farther away you are from hell, the closer you are to heaven.

No matter the personal challenges you face, you have to look for the good things in life and accept the ups and downs as they come along. I have had one of the most rewarding careers in the world, albeit complete with stressors more complex than those of other occupations. But when you have a positive attitude and people around you who are on your side, you can't lose. When your co-workers work as hard as you to help the people around you, it's a win-win situation even on a bad day.

I often felt blessed to be on the front lines of health care as an EMS provider. Only on a few days did I feel cursed, especially after witnessing the aftermath of a few great tragedies. But bad days help us to appreciate how precious life is. On most calls we got our patients to the local ER in a slightly better condition than how we found them. But on some days, our calls went to hell on route, no matter our interventions.

On scene, we were often presented with a traumatic or a medical disaster and, somehow, we figured out the best method of intervention regardless of the odds against us. The more calls you do, the better you become at problem-solving. We would assess the patient, interpret the complications, and then stabilize as best as possible, after which we would package the patients and get them into the back of our ambulance as quickly as possible. We would then make a mad dash for the closest or most appropriate hospital. We kept this up 24/7, 365 days a year, even when we were sick, tired, scared, and/or physically exhausted. Saving a life is the best way to recharge a broken spirit. One person with a positive attitude can help change everyone's day, and some days, we needed all the help we could get.

On good days, the patient survived the transport and they got a second chance to live. On our worst days, they died on scene or on route. Sometimes, we were unable to find or reverse the cause of the trauma in time for a successful outcome. No matter how good you are, sometimes destiny and fate can't be altered, despite a valiant attempt. It was not common, but it did happen from time to time. Losing a patient made me appreciate the saves even more; the fact that heaven needs good people takes the edge off a tragedy. Some days, it's all about the celebration of a person's long and wonderful life. No matter what people say or do in life, all life is precious.

If only we had the magical medical tricorder from *Star Trek* that could diagnose any medical condition in seconds! We could simply scan the patient and our diagnosis would be made. Decades of service attending calls makes one faster at diagnosing sick and injured patients. The fast scan and the serum lactate are the closest predictors of internal injuries and illness in our modern system. Technological advancements are never stagnant in our modern and diverse universe, and maybe there'll be a tricorder in my lifetime. It could happen.

Luckily, we can do a lot with our instincts and our current monitors, and experience is an effective substitute for Doctor McCoy. We would resort to our education, assessment skills, and ability to rapidly diagnose, and rely on our state-of-the-art Physio Control LP-15 to give us a patient's vital signs. We also had access to an on-line-medical consultant (OLMC) to give us directions. Some days it just came down to gut instinct.

We did our best, despite having limited diagnostic or laboratory equipment. We primarily went on our dispatch information but often it came down to the mechanism of injury and the patient's past medical history to try to come up with the best hypothesis of the primary medical concerns. We used our best educated guesses to treat the complications we could see, and we prayed for improvements in the patient's presentation or their vital signs. If their level of consciousness improved, we knew we are at least heading in the right direction with our care. If they continued to deteriorate, we kept looking for the underlying problems and implemented our life-saving interventions. We never simply gave up. To give up was not an option.

We would often take a deep breath as we unloaded our patients and headed to the trauma room or the resuscitation room. There the hospital staff would swarm us, and our job would almost be complete. It was often after the transfer of care when we started the cleanup that we realized the seriousness of the call we had just been through. That's often when it hit hardest. Some days those feelings were overwhelming. It wasn't just the patient who had been affected; often there were many people involved in the calls or events. It's astonishing how many people can be affected by one call, from bystanders to first responders, EMS, police, firefighters and hospital staff—and the effects can be felt for some time to come.

No single rescuer saves people; it's a team effort. We shared the wins and we also shared the losses with our co-workers. It wasn't helpful to keep feelings bottled up inside. Working together meant looking after each other, even when we didn't see eye to eye. It was after we went home that bad calls could haunt us. You could never predict the reasons why they would negatively affect certain responders, but nobody was immune from their effects.

The effects of bad calls aren't usually seen right away, but multiple stressful events in a short time frame certainly add up. When we get home, and let our guard down, is when the harmful side effects become more evident. As first responders, we often see death, suffering, pain and a broken society and, somehow, we start to think it's normal when it's not. It's when we have time to break down specific events that the reality of the calls impacts our inner selves. While on shift, we let our defences block the reality of events until we are ready to deal with them. Sadly, too many situations all blend together. When we don't process events on a personal level, the events hurt us more over time.

The lost sleep, the worrying, the flashbacks, the nightmares, the difficulty functioning at 100% take a toll over time. A sixteen or twenty-four-hour shift can challenge one's endurance and limitations. On a bad day, one's perception of the world can be overwhelmingly negative, and it can be almost impossible to see the good things around you. The loss of co-workers and fellow EMS colleagues to suicide due to post-traumatic stress disorder (PTSD), and the affliction of countless others by compassion fatigue is more prevalent than previously realized. No matter how well you perform your magic of saving lives, there will always be certain calls that never really go away.

In the end, the repercussions from bad calls never do go away for some people. Caring, dedication and repeated exposure to terrible events can be a double-edged sword. It hurts us during and after the calls. Some people aren't affected as much as others and it is easy to see that everyone reacts differently. Some days you have it easy and some days your calls are bad or more difficult. Some staff simply have bad luck, and some have terrible luck when it comes to seeing tragedy and dealing with its after-effects. New graduates and seasoned paramedics are equally affected. My bad days were not unlike those of others, although over the years they added up.

For the record, we don't all want the calls that force us to use our advanced lifesaving skills or ALS medications every time we go out. I love the calls where we get to visit with patients. Often, they start telling you their personal history and forget their current suffering and pain. Love and caring truly decreases stress and help heal bad days. One thing they don't teach you in school is not to count the bad calls. Count the good ones and then subtract the bad calls and, in the end, you should have a positive number.

I learned that to combat the bad calls, you had to add up the good ones first. You needed to keep them in perspective. The bad ones still counted, but it gave you a better perspective on your professional self-worth if you looked your entire body of work clearly and fairly. We truly do make a difference.

We need to go to work prepared to help people; EMS is a profession where excellence matters. Not every day is a successful one, but we probably have a better than 95% success rate. A positive attitude is everything and worry is a waste of energy.

The tragedies we responded to were never planned or known in advance. It seemed that some first responders attracted bad calls more than other staff. Even though we didn't know the patients or anything about them, they mattered to us just as much as the patients we knew. The emotional attachment to someone who is hurt, injured or sick is unmeasurable, unconditional and almost magical. It is not something that should reasonably happen, but you can get attached to a stranger, and then you will fight for their health for no other reason but to win the fight against the "Angel of Death."

When you add the other parts of your private or personal life that matter on to your professional stress is when it can really become overwhelming. It's easy to say, "Don't take your work home with you," after your shift, but it's not that easy to just drop it off in the ambulance bay on your way out and forget the tragedies or the events of the day. We all need time to process events and store them in the proper location inside our brains. Then we can come up with the solutions and the healing needed. Often when you have had time to rest and let the pieces come together like a jigsaw puzzle, you can see parts of a call relived in slow motion, reminding you that it really did occur. Then it becomes even more real, but not always in a good way.

Many people have been placed in the world at just the right time and in the right position to help others. Just when you think everything is going right with the perfect job, the perfect home life, and the perfect relationship, things can deteriorate. The world around you can fall apart, and you can crumble. Your structure or support system fails, and your life comes to a complete halt. That's a reality of professions such as EMS, police, firefighters and the military that wasn't previously acknowledged, but the side effects can be very harmful. We are not immune to having a life crisis. We typically care almost too much for others, to the extent that we don't look after ourselves. We look after everyone around us first and then we try to care for what's left of us.

While working for more than thirty-five years, I was involved in many patients' personal and tragic situations. As a team of professionals, we simply did our best when we were called to help the sick and injured. At the end of the day, we walked away knowing that some days we just couldn't save or help everyone. I suspect that my reason for doing what I did was the same as that of my co-workers. I would have to say I lived to work, and I worked to live. Over the years, however, many things caught up with me. I experienced the side effects of post-traumatic stress disorder (PTSD) and compassion fatigue. No one is immune to a lifetime of hurt and pain. The pain and the desperation to make sense of it all, is not something you would wish on a mortal enemy.

After one too many bad calls and the repeated loss of lives that mattered, I became a victim of PTSD, as well. I blame the system for it, even if no one takes the credit. The patients and victims we see matter more to us than we can comprehend. We strive to perform miracles, when even a miracle is not enough. We hate to lose for any reason. We were never taught in school that losing is an acceptable or even a humane outcome in certain cases. When your patient is palliative, and they have had a good life, we are there to help them reach their destination with dignity and humanity.

Many times, we assume blame for bad outcomes even if they are not our fault. We focus on our failures when we should be celebrating the wins or the success stories, even when the outcomes were destined to fail from the very start. Dr Peter Brindley a very gifted critical care intensivist I know summed it by saying "We know what injuries or disease processes are compatible with life, and we also know which ones are not." Often it is a person in his position who must make the final decision regarding the withholding of care. Too often, we take these failures personally. Only with professional psychological help was it possible for me to see that simple, but obvious, lesson. We can't always make a miracle possible. Some battles had been lost before we arrived.

I believe that each one of us is placed on this planet for a specific purpose. When I see my co-workers at my side, I know this was the right profession for all of us. My motto is simply, "I am a caretaker and lifesaver." I draw breath from helping others. We all bear some stories we can't share easily. Some secrets are better left uncovered, for the truth will help no one.

Some days, I wonder how I made it this far as a paramedic, and I realize it's all rather complicated. In simple terms, we need to develop our own unique personality, then we need to grow professionally and personally to strengthen our mind and body. Most importantly, we need to adapt to our environment and learn to be resourceful.

If you look carefully, you will notice that destiny often makes our paths cross those of our patients for a specific reason. It's kind of strange to think about destiny as something we can alter, modify or outright challenge. But with the right training and the right interventions, used at the right time, we can alter many life-threatening and critical events. We can save lives together with our co-workers' support. We can lessen our own pain by letting others around us share our hurt and take away the burdens we accumulate on the calls that hurt us the most.

With this book, I will try to change destiny by providing people with the stimulation to change their own world, thereby affecting all of mankind directly or indirectly. The rest I will leave up to my students, co-workers and friends. If we leave the world better off than it was before we came along, it's a positive outcome. Remember that nothing we do for the good of others is a waste of time, even if our efforts are in vain and our patients don't have a fortunate outcome.

Our efforts soothe those left behind just by knowing that someone gave their loved one every chance to survive. We aren't meant to save them all, but that shouldn't stop us from trying. If we continually educate ourselves about our profession, if we work as a team for the right reasons along with the right attitude, anything is possible. We can ultimately make the world a better place. Together, our interventions and our patients' will to survive helps them to recover from their trauma and live a healthy life.

If you had seen me in my younger years I was nothing special at all. But inside I was more unique then you could imagine for a boy from a small-town community. Somewhere inside my larger-than-normal-sized head, there was a vision to change the world, and any bumps I faced along the way were just part of my journey. I learned a long time ago that we are in harm's way 24/7, 365 days a year in the EMS profession. It's a risk/benefit ratio on some days. Any call we respond to could be one where we have to risk our own life.

Over the years I've been repeatedly knocked down, hurt and broken, and I've been sutured up and emotionally scarred from some events. I never really realized until several years ago that there are invisible injuries from the mostly unknown and not wholly understood post-traumatic stress disorder (PTSD), as well as major effects from complex compassionate fatigue. Somehow it walked right past our defenses and took the lives of some very good people before we could figure out the ways to help manage the side effects of repeated exposures to very traumatic and unimaginable events.

In our profession, we have more to offer if we focus on doing our best. If we make it our goal to do the best we can, then the outcomes will be more positive. Nothing is worth anything unless it is done with honesty, endurance, integrity and effort, and it comes from our heart. Along the road of life, we should humbly walk but look around us so that we don't miss anything.

We must never disregard our personal lines of defence. We must constantly be vigilant of our surroundings. Danger is always just around the next corner, and we must be ready to react. We need to change our linear thinking and use our peripheral vision to remain safe. We need to learn to see things other people choose to ignore. We need to learn how to feel pain that others choose to not feel, and we need to intervene when others walk away. We only get one chance to make a difference. Working as an EMS professional is an art, and as you evolve you achieve higher levels of functioning.

A job in emergency medical services (EMS) is for people who care about others, who want to help others, and who need to see others succeed, often before attending to their own needs. There will be many days when we will not get our breaks, we won't get enough sleep, and we will give up our personal time for the benefit of others. We must choose to give others' hope, and to take over another's problems on a moment's notice, if for no other reason than because we can. As we progress through our careers, we must adapt and accommodate to the world, or we will fade out from the profession. If you refuse to change your mind, refuse to adapt your base of knowledge, or refuse to adapt to the new members in the profession, you have already decided your fate. You have jeopardized your future.

My success stories were never just mine. I always had help from partners or co-workers. I have been blessed with having had many remarkable partners. Most people would not believe the hell we have survived to get this far in this profession. I'm sure that many of you who are reading this book can relate. You all have your own horror and success stories that you can choose to share if the time is right and the audience worthy. I trust you'll take the opportunity to vent your frustrations when you are safe and with people you trust.

In this book, I will write about multiple people who have been a positive influence in my world. In some cases, the names are real, and in other cases, they are not. Some of the cases described are real events that happened in my life, and others are completely fictional. Many people have helped me face my worst days and have helped me to walk away, even if I was still hurting. The memories of saving or helping people are what keep me going.

It's amazing the influence that one person can have in helping you become a better person. We all have a specific role or a specific purpose in our life; even if we can't see it, someday it will be revealed. Never miss a learning opportunity when it comes your way. Never miss a chance to make amends for a mistake. Often our mistakes are due to a lack of wisdom resulting from lack of knowledge. I can honestly say I learned my share of lessons the hard way.

We are teamed up with our partners in EMS for a reason. Frequently, my partner has made me look better at the end of a long and hard day. I have always protected my partner throughout our shift and that is the way it always will be in my world, just as I know they will look after me. The magic of having the right partner lets us alter the destiny of others in ways not believed possible. Working with a partner and working as a team allows us to accomplish incredible feats that are difficult to replicate. It is humbling to look back at the roads we have all travelled to get to our ultimate destinations.

Nobody Walks Alone – Walk 2017

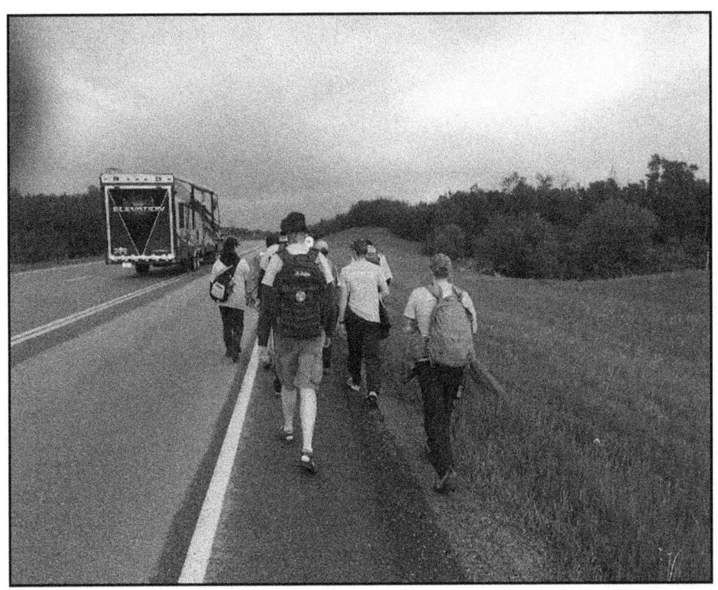

Thoughts for the Day

Every EMS team must have a leader.
Every EMS team must have a driver and an attendant.
By always working together, we can help each other.
When we work as a team we have the best chance of an improved outcome, despite facing some very devastating illnesses or injuries.
After the bad days, after the bad nights, just know you are still part of the same team.
After your shift, after a bad day, a friend is just one call or one text away.
When we walk along the EMS roads of life, we are never truly alone.
You are never alone if you choose to be part of the team.

The difficult days will be fewer if you let others help.
Don't ever give up.
Your pain is real.
Don't quit.
You're not alone.

Introduction: Changing the Future

Heather my EMS friend for life!

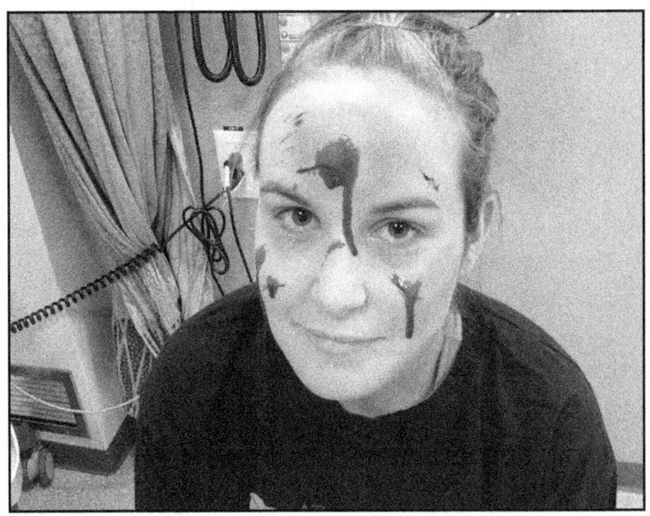

Life's best lessons start with us being the student

Life can teach us many lessons if we are willing to learn. The more I learned, the more I realized I knew nothing at all. For example, I learned, over time, that good people can come from bad situations and bad people can come from good homes or from good people. We cannot, nor should we ever judge anyone by their appearance. We need to take them at face value, at least until they prove their intentions. Most people are inherently good, even if they come off a little different than normal. Give them a chance.

We need to give others a fighting chance to make it on their own merits. We see people every day for whom the world has done no real favours. Many times, I see this in new students and new staff stumbling to make the best of their role. Often, they only lack a little outside guidance, a little mentoring to do the right thing, and then they make better decisions. We can stop what we are doing and look them in the eye and tell them we have their back. We can make them feel that they are part of the winning team.

A caring profession is not an easy one to walk into for we all have our walls and our defence systems for self-preservation and safety. We need to open our hearts to our new co-workers and welcome them in. They need to know they are in a safe place. We, too, were once students or new to a team in the past. Opening our hearts can get us in trouble some days when the ones we are trying to help turn on us or make fun of us. Many of us have let our defences down in the past and been hurt physically, mentally or emotionally. After we have been hurt by someone we cared for, it takes time to trust others on the same level again. But we slowly heal, and, in time, we come to realize that we were put on this world to make a difference. We just might hold our shields up a little higher when it comes to the next intervention. Some people might perceive that we are hard or bitter. Just know many of us were once burned or hurt by someone we thought we could help, and it makes us build protective walls.

The health care profession is very dynamic and complex. The essentials of what it takes to be an EMS professional are not combined in any single book. In our professional life, we all have a unique skill set that we develop and master to perform the art of keeping people alive. With our skills and our desire to help others, we have a purpose in life. We all need a purpose: to feel wanted, to feel needed or to have a reason to get up every day.

For us to get this far we have all seen our share of challenges, trials and tribulations. Those challenges make us stronger and wiser. With those challenges, we may make our share of misjudgments or errors. That's part of the career we opted to master. No matter who we are or at what level we practice, we all belong in the profession if we meet the minimum requirements. We have a role on the team, which is primarily to help people in need and to hopefully save lives even if we can't see or are not sure of our patient's life destination. As we mature in our role, we master our skills and, somehow, we make our lives more productive even if we have difficult or complex jobs. We overcome the changes as they challenge our normal days. Over time, we evolve into better people if we truly wish to belong in the circle of caregivers.

Many of us have spent years training, then spent years refining our art, and it's all put to the test as we arrive on the scenes of more complex calls. It is amazing how we expand our knowledge and adapt our treatments via education, training and the use of our intuition. Although we were taught how to help others, we were not taught the effects of the pain, the hurt, and the losses of life that we must face daily. The one part we can't seem to understand is the effect of the pain and suffering on us as first responders, even if we don't know or see the harm. We don't have a parent or a wise person standing by to tell us to be careful or to watch out for harmful situations which could affect our mind or body. Often, we don't have anyone to warn us about potential harm, so we learn to be more cautious with time and experience. The calls that bother us the most are multifaceted and can promote a certain fear of what may lie ahead. Our senses trigger alarms long before we go to the hard calls. But we go anyway.

The scene is always enhanced by the sounds, odours and emotions that are present at the time. After a call is over, we face the realization of the hurt and its aftermath on the broken people and the effects of a patient's injuries on our own lives. The blood all over our stretchers, our uniforms and the inside of the ambulance unit are evidence of the type of call it was. We find a yellow container that is meant for blood or bodily fluids and start to wash away the evidence of the call as soon as we can. On a good day, other crews or a good supervisor will show up and help us clean and restock our units, then we all work at making sure the task is completed. A good supervisor knows when to talk and when to listen. They know the type of pain and hurt we carry as they have seen their share of bad calls in the past.

The willingness of our co-workers or a supervisor to lend an ear or a helping hand are what we need on our bad days. It does us good to know that we matter and that someone cares enough about us to share in the cleanup. They have been in our shoes many times and they also know the effects that certain calls have on us all. I had many calls where after I went back to the unit, I almost cried looking at the destruction of our unit, the blood or body fluids all over, forcing me to accept the fact that the person we just transported was in a terrible position, often fighting for their life. Some days we lost the fight. The patient's life was over despite all our valiant efforts.

We often get called to situations that we know are bad from the start. Our dispatch information often prepares us ahead of time for the chaotic scene that awaits us. We start to prepare ourselves mentally and physically, and we adapt our bodies to be ready to tackle any intervention, so that when we arrive we are ready for the battle of a lifetime. It's often then that we realize that our battle is one that is going to be hard to win. You need to know and need to realize that, sometimes, only with divine intervention can some people be saved. We have all seen miracles or outcomes that are way beyond our calling as paramedics or as EMS staff. I would say it's divine intervention, regardless of your beliefs or your level of understanding of religion.

Some days, you just can't shut off your efforts to maintain an airway, sustain breathing, or continue ongoing treatment modalities to maintain circulation. These are the ABCs of patient care which we rely on to eliminate mortal threats as we progress throughout the call, even as we roll into the trauma room. In many cases we aren't even done doing everything we want to do when the physicians, nurses, and allied health staff take over and our battle to save a patient's life is turned over to them.

After we gave our verbal report to the hospital staff, we would grab our equipment and our stretcher and then head back to the unit to grab the ePCR or start cleaning up the mess. The attendant normally completed the ePCR and the driver started the cleanup process. We would sometimes go look through the back doors of our unit and be greeted by a surreal vision: blood on the walls, the ceiling, the equipment bags. A camera never did a bad scene justice, as it needed to be seen from multiple different perspectives to fully understand it. Then the next bad call would usually be not so bad. No two calls were ever the same. Every call was a learning experience if you took the time to reflect on it, if you took the time to evaluate what went well and what you could do better in the future.

To be successful in EMS, we learn to function in our assigned roles but, more importantly, we learn to intermingle with others for a specific reason. We are part of a larger team and we need to support them just as much as they support us. We all interact with the world at different levels; that is, we all offer a unique skill set but we only have a limited amount of time to make a difference in the lives we touch. For each of us, the time we spend with our patients is different, and there is no guarantee of tomorrow for anyone. We need to take the time we have and use it wisely in any way we can help or reach out to others. It is often after an unsuccessful cardiac arrest call that we appreciate the fact that time is valuable even more. You don't need training or skills to care.

We can show others what it takes to make our profession better by being a mentor or a positive role model. I challenge every one of my past students to carry on this legacy. At the end of the day, if we learn to work as a team and we help others have a better outcome, then I'd say it is a worthy profession, despite the battles or the hardships we must endure to make it to the other end of the roads we travel. We will have bad days. But our patients and their loved ones will have much worse days than we will, and that is a lesson you will need to learn on your own. The EMS world is not all about the adrenalin rush or being allowed to drive fast. If you can program your brain to go to work and have a good day, you will be happier. To always look for the good in the world around you is a great start.

After sitting and thinking about our global EMS system, I came up with the idea to describe the ideal EMS system in a book. Such a book could help to set the foundation for a future EMS service with many enhanced functions and staff abilities to help our profession evolve. In this book I will cover the essential requirements for such a system, such as the challenge of providing a higher level of care. I will show others how we can make the best of our services with nothing more than a desire to succeed. I will also take you on a journey of what it takes to become an EMS professional: the training required, the mental, physical and personal requirements. I want to share our profession with anyone interested in what we do. Hopefully, we can influence the next generation to join our profession.

At my best friend Ann Marie's funeral, I got the simple but clear message that "life is but a test." Living, or how we live life, is just a challenge and we can't get out alive but what we do while we are her on this earth defines if we pass the test. This book is a work of fiction but throughout it are woven years of wisdom, caring, compassion and personal inspiration from real events. It's my humble opinion that we should never do anything we think is wrong or that is not in our scope of practice. This book is was spawned from the many educational and difficult events I experienced over my career. Many lifelong lessons come from past tragedies that become inspirational, paradigmatic events.

Over the years, I have realized that certain people are meant to succeed in this world while others are doomed from the very start. Most of our life unfolds as it is meant to be unless we challenge our destiny. I'm going to challenge destiny like few others. I'm going to help my many students become leaders. I'm going to help my partners continue the legacy of helping others by simply doing the most logical and caring thing possible. We will collectively show the world we are a positive force against the forces of nature that are often working against us. There is good and there is bad in this world. We need to stay as close to the good side as possible to leave the world a little better off than it was before we came along.

My dream to help our EMS family is growing and is possible . . . We are walking for all EMS, Police, Fire Fighters and First Responders.

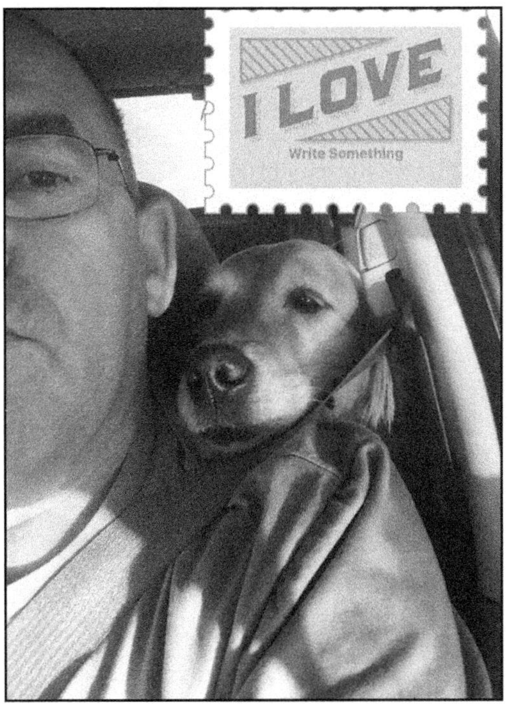

#NoOneWalksAlone2018

Chapter 1: Returning to the EMS World

"One More Challenge"

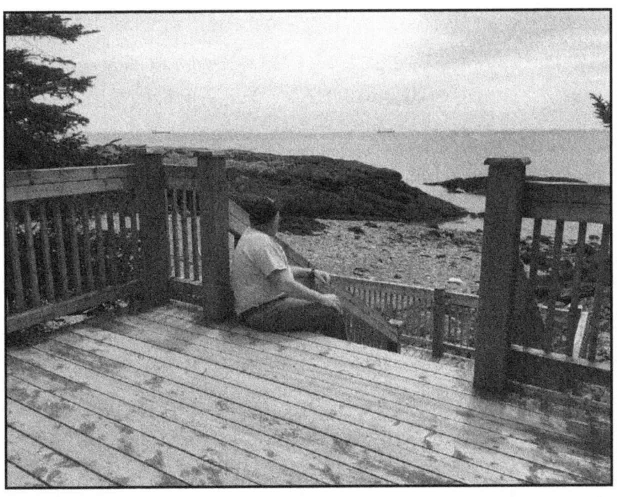

Facing life's' biggest challenges takes the support of all our friends

There was a time that I thought I would never be able to go back to emergency medical services (EMS) or stay in health care for any reason at all. But after a semi-working holiday, working the odd shift just to keep my skills current, my desire to go back to work started to grow. It's so hard to retire when it's such a big part of your life. I guess somehow my fate and my destiny were about to change even if I had no idea the EMS world was not done with me just yet. I thought about it long and hard and I had to know if I had one last push in me to try and change the world. I believed that if I was working full-time in a good organization it was possible. But I also knew life had knocked me down and hurt me badly in the past. It was the mental and physical challenges that many can't see and that you can't predict that did me in. An inner fear of failing, perhaps a fear of letting others down or getting lost along the way was all too real. I couldn't go back and face failure.

Once you have seen hell, it's harder to go back again, even if it is what you were meant to do. The fact that you were affected by post-traumatic stress disorder (PTSD) and made it back says lots, but the simple fact remains that you are never quite the same. Many people don't see or understand mental health issues or the cumulative effects that wear on your body. I know the past can and will haunt me at unpredictable times. We can't prevent the bad calls from being stacked against us. All we can do is be ready to face them and have a way to reach out for help when it is needed, and then simply just do our best.

I didn't know if I had any fight left in me to make a difference, but I knew I had a few people around me who could keep me going. I was determined I could and would help change the future of others, even if it was on a small scale. I woke up one day and I had dreamed of a better system and the dream just would not die. It was enough that I knew I had to try one more time. Even if it killed me, I was going to fight my last battle with integrity and honesty, and if I went out, it would be on my terms. Then I could finally walk away and hold my head up high despite the world falling apart around me for so many different uncontrollable reasons. You need to pick the battles you can win or that are worthy of fighting. My personal fight to help people was a battle I could win.

Many of the current EMS problems are beyond any of our abilities to control or change. I dreamed of a preventative strategy, a team effort and a way to change to become a progressive EMS world. With active community involvement, the prevention of accidents and illness would be a great accomplishment, instead of always being reliant on the actions of first responders. I dreamed of our younger generation changing the world by helping each other in times of an emergency. Our only hope was for our community members and our children to want to change the world. With the participation of EMS professionals, we could help build a remarkable service unlike any other in the world.

After meeting with the right people, I had a job; it was only a term position, but it was a start. I asked if we could have a round-table discussion to brainstorm ways to make our EMS system better than it was, in its current state. I guess someone wiser than me had bigger plans for my life, but I wanted to retire knowing we had the best system possible in place. I wanted the people I admired and trusted with my life to have a better system. I was fortunate, as I had seen the service from its birth through its changes, and at the end of the day the job was the same, just more complex.

My current supervisors knew I was very passionate about change for the right reasons. I just wished that if I made a plan that could be achievable, someone would see my dream and follow the steps needed to make it a reality. Somehow, we could make our service the best community paramedic service and become a new leader in our profession. Our children and our young people could become leaders in changing a broken society. We needed the basics of standard first aid and cardiopulmonary resuscitation (CPR) to be mandatory in our junior highs and high schools. Our children need to know the effects of the hazards and dangers of the real world. They needed to be able to make informed choices. They needed to matter in our community. They need to be prepared to eventually assume the leadership of our modern world.

With the right staff, we can be a positive influence on our communities. I'd seen some very good staff and some not so good staff come and go from our past services. As with every service, management had its good and bad points, but the current structure needed an overhaul if we were to make the system sustainable. At the end of the day, we need a community-involved EMS system staffed with essential workers. If you want the best employees, you need to ensure that you have the rewards needed to keep them. The money was part of it, but positive working conditions, along with a positive atmosphere are mandatory to the success of the service. Personal pride from the staff makes the service better in many aspects.

Every province has a different EMS structure with different skill sets and unique service requirements depending on their service location. Although we all try to model the national level when it comes to emergency medical responder (EMR), basic life support (BLS) and advanced life support (ALS) services, the services are all very different. In our province we have contracted and non-contracted services, both of which operate under different rules. I'm not against private operators or a provincial system, but I hate seeing different rules for different systems. I thought about the biggest problems over the weekend, and then decided that a better system was possible, but only if we build it from the ambulance base and expand it across the community. It needs to be what is best for the people, as well as what is best for the communities, and it must be practical and financially feasible to be maintained.

We needed a global change to the whole system. I was not willing to make suggestions or plan a new system if I thought I was wasting my time and effort. In my dream of an ideal system, we would amalgamate Fire, EMS and the educational system. We would incorporate the active first responders, emergency medical responders (EMR) in our modern EMS world. We would find a way to make our society safer, more accountable, and we could help prevent premature death and preventable injury when it was at all possible. We would ensure equal access to advanced life support (ALS) even in the more remote communities. We would need to work as a team and not remain a multi-tiered EMS system. We needed to respond as a team, and transport patients with a team mentality.

If we were to change, we needed to get the buy-in from management, as well as from community leaders, local schools and associated staff to help make our involvement worthwhile. Eventually, we would need the local medical overseers to help us change our service to one with an expanded scope of practice. With the Health Professions Act legislation, that was not going to be such a difficult process, as we could slowly increase our service if we had controlled and logical processes in place to make it work. With the right education, protocols and accountability, we could enhance the service to be the best in the world.

So, the first step was that I had to find the right people for the team and we had to plan this right from the start. I knew who I needed without a question. I needed to work with some of my past primary care students to mentor them, and I needed Sarah to return, as she was graduating as a paramedic soon. I could mentor her for the first several months and make her better than anyone I had ever worked with in my whole career. If we had a chance to work as a team again, we could change the world. I called them, and they immediately said "yes," and my heart restarted. Now we had a chance to change the world. With the right team and pure determination, anything was possible. Together, we would make it work and then I'd retire and make my way east. I would be packed, in my truck and headed about 4500 kilometres east to make a new home for the rest of my years. Pebbles and my new dog Ember would be at my side and we would be moving on. That was the plan that would make my life fulfilled.

Thinking back, I honestly don't know how it was possible to be in the emergency medical services (EMS) field for so many years. I just kept doing casual work to keep me from going insane. But I needed the stimulation and patient contact to stay alive. I had no idea I was going to get a chance to come back and try to change the system one more time. I knew Sarah, my old partner, could get me through it for she was my angel, and with the help of a few others we could make the EMS profession take a step ahead and not back.

I worked shift work for many years and went on many difficult calls. For many years, it seemed like the local service always ran short-staffed. Add to that a super-high call volume, a high acuity of calls, as well as many mentally and physically challenged calls, and it took a toll on all of us. Then, unfortunately, some staff were injured or needed extra sick time. Somehow, the local EMS services never stopped working; in fact, the calls just increased from year to year, and the calls became more complex.

Staff were being pushed harder and harder, both mentally and physically, and for many, the breaking point was just around the next corner. I wanted to find a way to take the pressure off the staff and share the responsibility of patient care among the community and the first responders, as well make the emergency medical responder (EMR) role more productive. I had a chance to change destiny, but it would take some imagination. With imagination, experience and intuition, a new idea was born for the next era of emergency medical services.

We all know we have a breaking point, but what we often don't know is what it takes to get to that breaking point. Every person has many unique and personal strengths that make the breaking point stay at least a few calls away. Looking back, the breaking point for our service was when it became apparent that staff were unable to respond to one more emergency call. But if we waited for that to happen, it would be too late to fix the problem. We were constantly pushing ourselves to the limit and using other resources to fill in when we were not able to respond. For example, we were increasingly relying on volunteer firefighters to take our medical calls. There had to be a better way, and this was my final chance to make the system better by doing it my way. I also thought a little more about our role in prevention and public education. The possibilities were endless, but the dream needed to be formulated, crafted and made a reality.

One's destination is where the heart takes you!

Chapter 2: Building a New EMS System

"The Best EMS System"

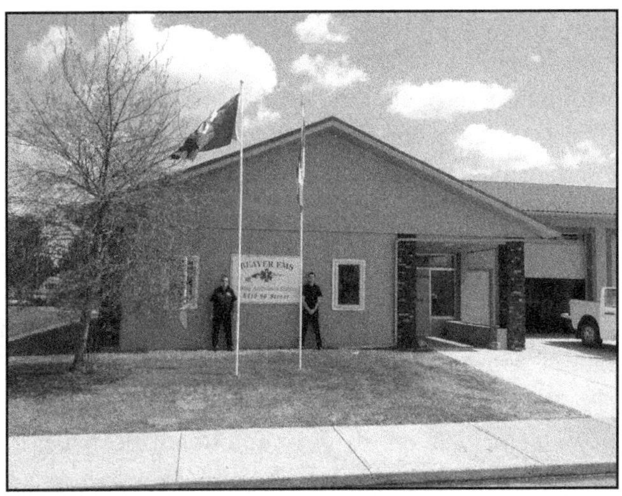

The right people on the team only make us stronger!

The initial plan called for me to work on the units for two tours of forty-eight hours on and six days off, then to see what worked and what needed to change. I would be buddied with different crews, as well, so I could see several different perspectives. There were three crews working and taking turns responding to calls, and every crew had a primary care paramedic (PCP), formerly known as an EMT, as well as an advanced care paramedic (Paramedic) on every call. Based on qualifications, the most experienced staff would qualify for the critical care paramedic (CCP) status. I would work to have multiple staff certified at the CCP level. Many of the staff already had the skills and had taken the required courses but needed formal certification. There are a few of them I'd trust with my life and the lives of my children and know they were being taken care of by the best of the best. They were truly gifted.

So, looking ahead we could change the world—even if it was just our own little world, we could and would make it better. We would be the best and most efficient EMS team in the modern world. Then I wondered: What if I could get the First Responder course into grade nine and grade ten classes and the Emergency Medical Responder (EMR) course into grade eleven and grade twelve classes? We could make a difference in the kids and younger adults! I had to think of a global change and not just a small change. I wanted our newest members to start as children or teenagers. I also wanted to encourage our society to educate themselves in, at a minimum, standard first aid and cardiopulmonary resuscitation (CPR), as a requirement to drive a car or to ride a pedal bike. There is so much we can teach to a younger generation who can easily absorb the material. At the end of the day, I just wanted children to know that street drugs kill and that everything in the real world has good and bad outcomes. No one drug, or amount of alcohol, is benign. Let's make our children be the future educators of society. We need them to be the ones to say this is wrong and thus save a life.

The day I went back to work started as per usual: we had three simple emergency calls and then we were called to assist in a BLS inter-facility transfer. At about 1500 hours, we were called to back up a basic life support (BLS) unit that needed help during an inter-facility transfer. I wondered why they had used a BLS unit in the first place when their service had ALS units available. This transfer was clearly an ALS transfer, as the patient had been in a significant motor vehicle collision (MVC) and internal injuries were suspected. This is a good example of our health care system's weak spots, and the patient and community were the ones suffering. Someone had let the system lose today. Either the sending physician was uneducated in trauma care, or the dispatcher was uniformed of the real situation. On top of it all, the crew was new and uneducated in the system, but thankfully they realized they were in trouble and called for ALS assistance.

In my eyes, ALS should be for everyone, especially in rural locations. Why do we use BLS when ALS is available? It was the one question I could not answer. We would cover for our co-workers' educational deficits and not set them up for failure. We should not put a new EMR and a brand-new primary care paramedic in such a difficult situation. We would gladly volunteer to do the transfer. We would volunteer to help get the people that need ALS care out of harm's way. Slowly, we could fix the broken system. With the spread of ALS courses to small rural hospitals, the care would improve.

My blood pressure went up about thirty points when my partner looked at me and told me to start an IV, and I realized they were sending a serious patient with no IV access, by a BLS crew for a computerized tomography (CT) scan. One would think that if a patient had a significant mechanism of injury (MOI), an ALS service or crew should be utilized. But as with many things, common sense does not always prevail in the medical world. So, we started from the top and did a head-to-toe assessment, applied a set of IVs, administered some pain relief, and added the CO2 monitor to assess ventilation and perfusion, and we were off. Now we needed a trauma centre with a trauma team, and not just a CT scanner.

Over time, a logical and shared system would only influence surrounding systems. We could make a state-of-the-art system that was second to none. We just needed the right people as leaders, support staff, and team members. Along with the right equipment and attitude, we could make miracles happen. With time, we could enhance all our roles and have something to be proud of for years to come, like the Squad 51 fire halls from the show *Emergency* (which for many of us was the real birth of the first paramedics in the early 1970s).

We assisted in the stabilizing of the patient and after a quick phone consult with on-line medical control (OLMC), we had a new plan of attack. We diverted the patient to the most appropriate location and ensured the patients care was optimal, despite the initial lack of care due to a flawed system. As we were a three-man unit (the advanced care life unit, as commonly referred to by paramedics), we all just jumped in their unit with our ALS kits and essential equipment, such as medication and IV pumps, thereby making their unit the ALS unit. We provided the extra help they needed with our primary care paramedic (PCP) in our unit following our every move down the busy highway toward the awaiting trauma team. We had some work ahead of us, but we would stabilize the patient and the outcome would be improved.

As we pulled into the ambulance bay at the trauma centre, I knew we had done a great job. The situation was stable, and the patient had a better chance all around. On arrival, the trauma team was more than happy to take over our critical patient. Ironically, despite our fluid bolus and care, the patient's lactate level (which tells us the severity of injury or damage) was over six (normal is less than two), signifying that no matter what we saw on the outside, there was serious injury inside the patient. The moral of the story is that the mechanism of injury (MOI) matters. The point is that we need more ALS mentors working the streets and doing the calls, instead of micro-managing from an office. We need ALS and critical-thinking medics on the street. We need community paramedics out in the communities. We are only as strong as our weakest link of prehospital care providers.

Thankfully, we were well-received in the receiving facility despite being rerouted from the original transfer destination. The trauma specialist ensured us he would provide feedback to our neighbouring service management as well as to the sending hospital to make sure that such an event occurred less frequently. The trauma team rapidly took over the care and we just had to finish our documentation and ensure the BLS staff were okay before we left them to return to their respective bases. They were very thankful, and we ensured that they knew we could help them anytime and they had our number if they had any questions.

All in all, it was a good learning opportunity for everyone. As we were walking out, our patient was already more stable, and the outcome was much more positive despite the poor start. Thankfully, the situation never became worse, or we all would have looked bad in the eyes of the family and with the public. Nothing looks worse than a patient dying in the back of a BLS unit while the ALS unit is watching TV or relaxing while getting paid to help but not being allowed to provide care.

As we walked out of the trauma hospital, our unit was waiting for us with our preferred Timmy's coffee at the ready for us. That is a true sign that you are a team. Everyone thinks about everyone else and ensures everyone is treated as well as possible despite the hardships we face from time to time. I gave our faithful and efficient PCP a high five and we both offered to drive the other home, but she won out in the end. I jumped in the back to a little protesting from the senior paramedic, but I told them today I was just a student of EMS life. On the way back, we discussed the common concerns we see in the present system and brainstormed ways to make our system better in time to come.

There is no perfect system. Even with good intentions, we can fail. Many years ago, we did an ALS/BLS intercept when critical care was needed. We were a dual ALS team that night because I was just riding along for fun. We planned to meet on the highway with the intention of carrying on to the most appropriate hospital after we assessed the patient's status. Our new PCP partner was the driver that night and he watched us jump into the BLS ambulance and I guess he didn't understand our plan of attack. He thought his job was done, so he turned the ambulance around and went back to our base after we had jumped into the back of a BLS unit, despite the fact that most of our ALS equipment was still in our unit. We tried to call him, but he had turned his radio down too low to hear our call for help. He was a very new staff member, so he didn't know the most important rule was to always stay right behind us and make sure we all get home safe. He never turned his radio to low again after that day.

After we got the patient to the most appropriate hospital we got a ride back to our base with the BLS crew. We all ensured this little error would not happen again and the new PCP was truly embarrassed. He would not leave us stranded on any highway or street corner again. From then on, he closed the back doors and tapped twice to let the driver know to get going. Just a simple lesson for us all that common sense is not always common. Many of our skills and interactions are learned behaviours. Just know it's never bad to clarify plans with everyone to make sure the team is all on the same page. Communication is of utmost importance, and it is never silly to ask any question to ensure everyone is on board. There are no silly questions in our EMS world.

Somehow, we had to try change the system, but first we needed to know what was broken in our own system or needed to repair what was broken locally to make our system better. I knew we could not fix the other systems, as they didn't or would not want to improve, until the staff forced the change. Positive changes would not happen unless the right leadership overcame the deficiencies or fixed the broken system from the top levels and worked downwards to fix it.

After the call was over, we had an open and honest debate, and settled on a few important guiding principles. Providing the highest level of care was our biggest priority. The number of staff members had to be increased, and they needed more frequent access to additional mandatory training. Extra staffing was also needed for education and community involvement, as well as the addition of more units to ensure our local community was looked after first and foremost. I thought we needed to poll the staff (especially the new staff) on a one-to-one-basis to hear what they felt were strengths and weaknesses in our service. Anyone found with a negative attitude concerning positive changes would be provided with encouragement to find a job someplace else. It always shocked me how a small group of people were never happy and seemed to thrive off negativity.

After we got back to the base, I started to talk to the staff on shift. I confided in the students about my personal mission on the current shift and asked for a few minutes of their time. I figured, if you needed to fix a problem, you should look to the newest, most junior, staff and work your way up. It was all about our perspective; an outsider has a unique take on our personal strengths and weaknesses.

I asked them what made this a good place to do a practicum and what made it not so good? "If you were me," I asked, "what would you do to help you be the best you can be?" I was not shocked by their answers, but in some cases, I was sad to learn the truth. I thought I would first try to focus on five good and as well as five bad points from our meeting and then go from there.

Five positive points that were made:

1. *Ours was an ALS service and we were very busy. For students, that made the learning much more real and sometimes more intense. It was helpful for students to understand call management and learn how to prioritize assessments and treatments, as they could practice it over and over to get better. After multiple calls they mastered their new role.*
2. *For the most part, students had more practice doing skills at the local EMS service than they ever had in the short time at school. One student came from a class of seventy-plus students. Thankfully, another student said they had lots of practice as the class was smaller and the instructors ensured that skills were performed in a supervised format, at least three times, which was good to know. So, as a mentor of students' equipment*

training, a review was deemed mandatory for every staff and every student.

3. *The best preceptors are the ones who want to mentor the students. The best mentors spent extra time with each student before, during and after a call, and went above and beyond by providing extra experience, extra training and constantly providing constructive feedback.*
4. *The use of teamwork is mandatory for better patient outcomes. For example, a paramedic working with the PCP and discussing openly back and forth what they had to do on every call is much more conducive to holistic patient care and also makes for a much more comfortable working environment. It needs to be a team effort.*
5. *When the preceptors took on a student willingly and made them feel like one of the team from the first call and ensured it was a quality learning experience, the experience was much more positive. More importantly, when all the staff took a role in helping the student, the student excelled.*

Five negative points that were made:

1. *When the preceptor was rude, condescending and uncaring toward patients, other staff or toward their job, the learning experience suffered. One student was pulled from a prior learning experience by their school facility as the staff were nasty and set the student up to fail from the very start. It made me sad to know that people could be so nasty in what should be a caring and therapeutic environment.*
2. *The EMS base is not very conducive to learning, when there is no opportunity to rest between calls and lack of nourishment over the course of busy shifts. Some days you don't get a break, and being on the go for sixteen hours straight is hard on anyone, even the experienced and most dedicated staff members.*
3. *Preceptors who expected the school to provide all the initial hands-on training and were not willing to help a student learn make for a negative experience. Often a student would have*

to find other staff to augment their learning deficiencies to be successful.

4. *Students were sometimes subjected to unreasonable expectations, such as not being allowed to sleep or to relax along with the regular staff. This is disrespectful toward our future co-workers.*
5. *Expecting students to manage complex calls right from the start is completely unrealistic. Once a student has become experienced at call management and feels comfortable in their role, they can be expected to delegate, manage and provide the appropriate care when it is requested. But to walk into a disaster is hard on even the most experienced staff, so to expect a student to be successful in such a situation is not reasonable.*

Overall, the most important lesson was that we needed for all staff to understand that, once we accepted a student, we needed to plan for that student's success. It was the responsibility of every person within the service to make the student's learning environment better. We also needed to work on a better training environment, a scheduled in-service method that worked for all staff and a better relief system for the busy crews. We needed an atmosphere that was conducive to learning, resting, sleeping when it was not busy, and we needed more staff and additional units. But for all this to happen, we needed the right team, from the student all the way to the management. I needed to work with the people in charge to plan such a global change. We needed to set up a timeline to work on the changes needed to make the progress trackable and accountable at all levels, by everyone involved.

The biggest component of change was to get "buy-in" from the current EMS community. The people from the community had to support the increased level of service, as did the supervisors and the current staff. Staff who were not willing to participate or unwilling to change, would not be optimal for long-term employment in such an EMS industry. Some would say they were burnt out, but I would argue that they were never meant to last. I think the phrase "burnt-out" and "in it for the wrong reasons" are two different things. With optimal selection criteria, training and resources, the strain on health care workers would be lessened. We also had to ensure we had adequate educational opportunities in place to ensure that all staff could increase their knowledge, especially as medicine is a constantly evolving field. If we are stimulated to evolve, to always be updated with the most modern skills and to have access to modern equipment that works well in our environment, our jobs become less complicated.

We all needed to help enhance our standard level of care. This went way beyond BLS, and was more complex than ALS care, and if we did it right, we would be the new leaders in the EMS world. The on-call quarters, the training room and the enhancements to the base would make the service much more attractive to potential staff in the future. But I had to ensure that I could participate at 110% in this role for my final EMS career. For my dream to be possible I needed the right people at my side and then all things were possible.

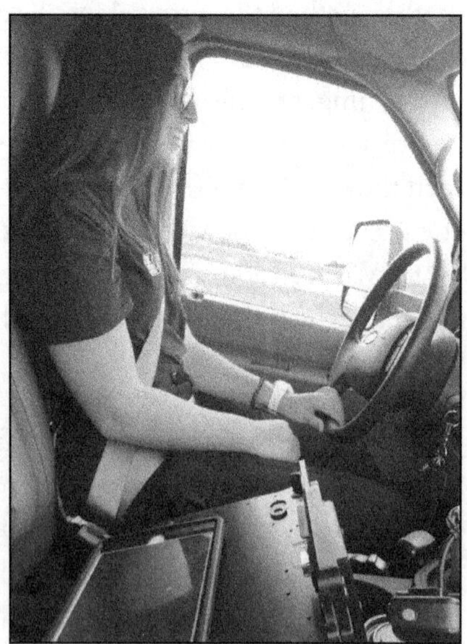

Nobody walks alone if we care

Chapter 3: Raising the Bar

"The Right People"

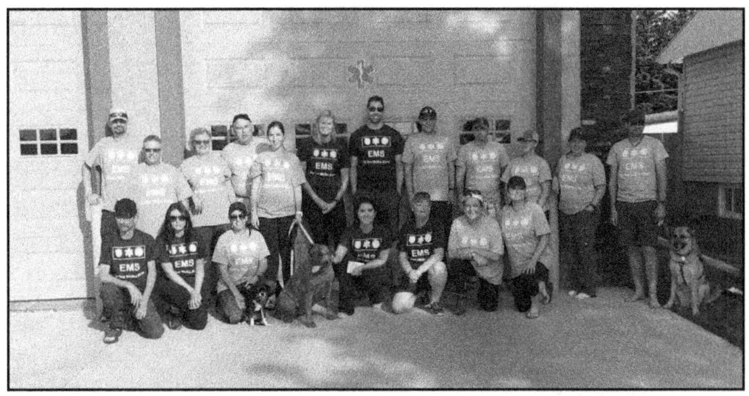

Nothing is impossible with the right people!

A proper station is one of the most important things an ideal EMS system can offer its employees. But much more than just the right building is needed for the system to work efficiently. It needs to be part of the community, to be responsive to the community's needs and to make a difference in the lives of the people it serves. Every community will have unique and different needs. The types of calls and their ensuring responses will vary from service to service. It stands to reason that we can take on a new student, bring them into our service and, in no time, make them one of our own. A great system is one in which people strive to ensure they are the best they can be and others strive to join them. The better the staff, the better the service, and thus the better the help that the community members will receive in times of need.

My dream was to ensure we had the right staff, right location and the right response system, along with the right base to work out of. My vision of the ideal team involves a basic life support (BLS) system working within an advanced life support (ALS) system. By employing primary care paramedics and advanced care paramedics working as a team, every patient would be entitled to BLS care on all calls and ALS when it was required. If you cover all the BLS aspects of a call, and then just add ALS skills, as required, you increase the odds of missing essential steps along the way. The more you practice, the better you will be. The more education you receive throughout your life and the more you maintain your competence, the more you will excel in your profession.

I reflected on the current system after working two weeks on both shifts and decided if we could shoot for the stars, even if we only hit the moon, we would still be better off than before we started. My biggest priority was a better EMS base, additional staff and units. Additional units that responded to better serve our patients and our communities and provided essential backup to our co-workers and allied EMS providers. We are not alone; almost every service could expand their EMS model and make the service better.

First, we really needed the right supervisors. We needed to ensure we had a leader who would be able to supervise off-car but still able to assist in all call management concerns. We would provide them with a rapid response vehicle to assist with medical emergencies and to support our units in times of need at emergency calls. A paramedic response unit (PRU) would be perfect for the supervisors. They were needed when something big happened or when we needed them to step in and take over. It was almost like having a real, live guardian angel built into the system.

Another important role every service required was a training officer. If it was my new role, I too would need to be up on the most modern treatments, medications and emergency medicine trends. We needed to actively try to reduce the negative outcomes within our emergency medical services profession. By working with staff and including them in overall care and by enhancing educational requirements, we could strengthen our team effort. We are accountable and required to be reactive to situations as they arise, so we needed to ensure our education was well-rounded and that we were able to rapidly adapt to any situation.

We needed to be supported before the call, during the call and after the call was completed. I wanted to ensure my co-workers always had a better system to fall back on when they needed it the most. I wanted our service, our community and our surrounding communities to have the best care providers in the world, following the model of emergency medicine fellowships in teaching hospitals. I believe that education needs to be cyclic, enhanced, always in touch with the current trends and standards, but also enjoyable and applicable to real life.

I would have to get some help to make this work. We would need management support. Our budget would have to be increased for additional units, as well as for staff. By providing a supervisor with a response vehicle to enable them to roam the community, it would make for better community support. Other co-responders would also be able to fill in for emergency staffing needs if a staff member got hurt or if a crew needed help to complete a call.

Our local EMS needs were changing, with the emergence of tactical EMS, palliative care and home care demands, and public education. The extra units were easy to justify but currently there was no place to park them and we needed the building for other purposes. The biggest problem was transitioning from the current base until we had the room to make it all work. My dream was to lean more on our volunteer staff. One idea was to have volunteers on our units to help train our local fire-and-rescue personnel. It stands to reason that it is only fair to train the volunteers we use. They could be our third person on the unit. At the top, we needed an educator to help to train our staff and volunteers, and more importantly, we needed to educate children in junior and senior high schools.

The one thing we could not truly gauge was the needs of the surrounding communities, but if our current and recent calls were any indication, we would be getting busier. There are many times that rural services are pulled into urban centres to help respond to calls, as the urban system is not meeting their current call needs. The most common concern was after we had completed a transfer from rural to urban and had pushed clear, we were often then placed into the urban hub of someone else's needs. Our rural centres went without or had to rely on other services to cover for our absence. Instead of being able to head back to home base to restock, recharge and to catch up on other daily tasks. On some days, that didn't happen until we timed out after sixteen hours on shift.

Our needs were more complex than outsiders could know. Ideally, the changes we needed or wanted were:

1. ***Additional ALS units, stocked and identical to our current units.***
2. ***Extra staffing for additional ALS unit.***
3. ***An additional BLS transfer unit for non-acute transfers (e.g. appointments, medical referrals to non-acute care centres, etc.).***
4. ***Supervisors for life support equipped with rapid response vehicles and renamed paramedic response units (PRUs).***
5. ***Staff for base duties (e.g. stocking and cleaning units).***
6. ***Educational officers for our staff, local schools and for community involvement and education.***
7. ***Community paramedics for community responses.***
8. ***Tactically-based EMS-trained staff equipped with a vehicle.***

After carefully looking at our community, it was easy to see that there were many more needs than we were currently addressing. We had always been in a reactive mode. Too much time and effort had been expended on fixing problems after fact, instead of learning from past mistakes and changing behaviours and engaging in prevention strategies. If we could reach younger generations and ensure they were trained and ready for medical emergencies at a basic level, it would be a start. Education remains the only way we can change the destiny of the children of tomorrow.

The initial requirement was to have all units equipped identically. It was an expensive yet essential requirement, and necessary so that staff could easily switch between any unit, assigned or otherwise. It was also important that the units be taken out of service post-call or post-shift to be cleaned and restocked. Quality control needed to be stringent in terms of mechanical, electrical and physical inspection to ensure that units were always ready to respond. After serious calls, we came back covered in blood or bodily fluids, our units are contaminated, and our stock had been eliminated. We tried our best to clean and restock after calls but, as with anything, there were times we forgot one thing or another. I've often found blood or other contaminants on items that were never even used. In an emergency, when multiple people are grabbing for equipment, things get moved or used, and one doesn't even realize it.

Extra staffing resources for an additional ALS unit would be a win-win for all of us. Many days we had calls back to back and we often needed extra time to clean, document, and restock the units. We would get by doubling up the equipment on board when possible, so that we could manage two serious calls back to back, but this was not ideal. An extra unit would ease the workload and we would be able to take units out of service to restock, clean and recharge the crews mentally and physically after difficult calls. After a bad MVC, a cardiac arrest, a serious traumatic event or any other complex medical call, the unit must be removed from service and returned to our base, cleaned and restocked. A unit check is advisable. There is nothing worse than going to another bad call and you're still short equipment as you haven't even made it back to base yet. We can't provide the best care if we are short on regular supplies or missing essential equipment.

An additional BLS transfer unit would be a good idea for some calls. Often, ALS units are booked for non-acute transfers for appointments or medical referrals to non-acute care centres, and there is no need to use either an ALS unit or a BLS unit. In some locations, a transfer unit equipped with a driver and an extra staff member would be ideal for such a task; moreover, it would be beneficial to keep an additional EMS unit in service. For example, I recall doing a twelve-hour transfer for a lady for a specialist ophthalmic appointment. It was a complete waste of health care resources, as an ALS unit was taken out of service for the duration of that transfer. Staff needed to ensure the transfer of patient care was not being abused. ALS staff needed to be able to decline non-essential transfers if a BLS or an ALS transfer presented. There is no ideal system, but there is hope for improvement. If only we did what was best for the patient at the end of the day we would have done the right thing.

Supervisors in rapid response vehicles needed the ability to flex between calls quickly, to provide backup or support to crews on scene and to assist with extrications. They could provide wisdom and moral support during difficult procedures; for example, a traumatic airway, a complete heart block, or a heart attack. Even though units are equipped with thrombolytic kits, patients are often very complex. An extra set of hands along with some wisdom can go a long way.

In the past, when it came to very serious calls, we were able to grab an extra set of hands and take off for the local ER or bypass to a trauma centre or a critical care centre. Ideally, we could simply call STARS air ambulance, but they can't fly in inclement weather and are often already tasked to a call. Currently, rural communities often dispatch the local fire service as co-respondents, simply because no other EMS units are available. As a consequence, the fire staff ends up in a short-changed position when responding to complex medical calls and are less prepared to handle them.

Base duties are more complex than many people take for granted. These consist of stocking, cleaning, staffing, training and constantly recycling stock from the units to the kits, then to the units. A certain selection of minimum stock supply must always be available. We can go for weeks without requiring certain equipment, and then we might require that equipment on three calls back to back. Staff for base duties, such as stocking and cleaning units, is essential. We need help to ensure the proper restocking and cleaning of units after calls. We often transport infectious patients who can easily contaminate staff and equipment if units are not cleaned properly.

The role of a supervisor is very complex and is not a job to be taken lightly. It needs to be filled by someone of integrity, with strong leadership abilities, and superior knowledge of our profession at all levels of care. A supervisor must be loyal to the service and willing to assume responsibility and ownership of their actions or lack thereof. A great leader knows when to lead and when to sit back and let staff perform their role. It's not a dictatorship when it's done right. A great leader leads by example, and their presence lends positivity.

The role of educational officer for staff is also often taken too lightly. The advancement and continual change in the emergency health services and medical technology dictates that EMS staff need to constantly be challenged and stimulated to enhance their practice. Communities and special populations dictate the educational needs of the staff. All staff have weaknesses, but these will vary among different levels of experience.

Any service needs to be aware of the population base which they serve, and the level and type of care required must be adapted to the people who need it. A community must consider populations who are more dependent upon extra care. The educational needs of any service must be adjusted to current and potential future needs of the population. As the health care system expands and changes, we need to adapt to the needs of the most vulnerable members of the community. The roles of the staff will trend to certain types of calls, such as medical traumas or emergencies. There will never be two services with the same type of call responses, transport times or challenges, due to geography or current health care structures.

Community needs can change in a short time because of unexpected local challenges. A good example is the current fentanyl crisis. Many people have been led to assume that Narcan is the solution, but they are dead wrong. It's not even an adequate bandage solution for the problem. To fix the problem, we must get to the root of it, such as why people do drugs in the first place. To achieve this, every service must adapt their services to meet the community needs and extra call volumes this epidemic has created. People can overdose more than once while one is on shift; if they are sent home, they can to do it all over again. The problem is not fixed.

The educational needs of any EMS service are constantly being challenged but are also cyclic. I wonder if the ideal way is the implementation of continuing education modules, or if it is cyclic reviews of the scopes of practice for all staff in a three to four-year cycle. The educational models of local schools could address integration of first-responder knowledge at various grade levels that would enhance community involvement. Training and resources could be provided for standard first aid and CPR in junior high and possibly for emergency medical responder (EMR) training in grades ten or eleven. This alone would elevate the level of future emergency care for an entire community.

Why not educate kids to be able to handle emergency events, to learn and understand the effects of disease and medication misuse on our bodies, and to have the ability to intervene at a basic level in medical or traumatic emergencies? It would be a great start to helping improve the health of our communities, to educate the generation that will affect the future.

Community Paramedics for Community Responses was a new adventure in urban centres, but less so in rural locations, due to a lack of funding and staffing and a dearth of people who understood the need for its inception. Its role was primarily to decrease a patient's visits to the local ER, thereby decreasing the burden on the health care system. Many services are available in the community, but not available 24/7, and especially not on weekends and on holidays. Often patients simply need assessment, followed by simple instructions, such as how to change dressings and what additional medications they may take, when it comes to regular medical and minor trauma care situations. There is also a need for resources for patients with behavioral issues, and for people who live on the street with no other means of access to health care.

Tactically trained EMS staff are present in major urban centres but less so in most rural locations. With societal changes such as the spread of drug labs, and the increase of rural crime, there's an ensuing increase in high-risk incidents involving the police in rural areas. We are in effect, letting bad guys get away with more and more, while the legal system is being taxed to extremes. EMS staff has to be available to assist the police in times of emergency situations such as drug-related offences, shootings or multiple victims in a hostile or dynamic scene. Staff need training in self-defense and in the protection of other allied health professionals in times of need. Tactical EMS basically covers stopping the bleeding, maintaining an emergency airway and getting the injured to safety.

Sadly, in times of economic shortages, provincial governments as well as hospitals tend to forego the importance of having a backup communication system. All too often, people forget the communication events that led to almost every local, regional, and provincial disaster in our lifetime. A backup system includes ensuring that communication is never lost in times of disaster. Past experiences show that the use of a cellular network is unreliable and thus not a stable platform for all situations. The use of VHF or UHF radio systems along with the provincial system ensures that there is always another form of communication available.

In an ideal EMS system, the ideal EMS base would contain:

1. ***EMS responding vehicles.***
2. ***Cleaning bays where units can be stripped, cleaned and restocked.***
3. ***Secure equipment/medication storage.***
4. ***Physical fitness and educational training rooms.***
5. ***Nutrition/entertainment room.***
6. ***Study rooms/dorm rooms for resting between calls***
7. ***Managers, support staff and a duty supervisor.***
8. ***Supervisor's office.***
9. ***Volunteer/community support room (public training room).***
10. ***Meditation or entertainment rooms where if you wanted to visit or just relax, it would be possible to do so with your co-workers. Somewhere you felt safe and that was away from the public and the busy side of the EMS base when you needed a break.***

After seeing many different bases, it was clear they were designed to cover the needs of the time, but expansion was seldom possible due to financial constraints. There is a lack of insight for future needs of the service, as well as for the expanding needs of communities. An ideal base would ensure that all EMS responding vehicles had a home and were stocked and ready to respond.

Any base needs to include cleaning bays where units can be stripped, cleaned and restocked. Many times, our bases have parking places for the units but no place to clean and restock them. We need a place where we can strip the unit of equipment, perform a deep clean and do an accurate inventory after our complex calls. Pride of ownership can certainly be seen when employees can maintain their units in ready condition!

It should be mandatory to have a well-lit place for the dispensing of medication that could also be used to secure expensive equipment. Staff must always be accountable for the security of medications. The environment must be temperature-controlled as certain medications cannot tolerate extreme temperature. Most importantly, there must be a system which allows us to track medication by lot numbers and expiry dates. Ideally, there should exist a warning by which medications are automatically reordered once minimal stocks are sensed.

A well-equipped physical fitness area, and an interactive training room for simulations and transfer practice and the like would be fabulous. It could be converted to an educational training for large groups or be able to be broken into multiple smaller stations for small group interactions. It goes without saying that bathrooms, showers and change rooms are a basic requirement. Proper nutrition can be challenging while on shift work. It is essential that a kitchen and eating area to be included in the plans. Many staff are trying to eat healthier, but it can be difficult to do so due to the duration and nature of unpredictable calls. Healthy snacks and fruit should be made available, in addition to a supply of portable (bottled) water.

Access to personal study rooms, dorm rooms with showers and private bathrooms, and for resting between calls is essential. Down time is important, but privacy in times of need is even more so. It is essential that shift workers take short breaks throughout their shifts to recharge. Some staff might be able and willing to power through a shift, but this is not the case for most people. When you do shifts back to back, your sleep cycle becomes altered and even a short break can recharge you for hours.

It's nice to have managers, support staff and duty supervisor's available in the middle of an operation. They also need privacy from the noise and daily functions of the service, the units and crew to be productive. A good service can run without management intervention, but it's important that staff and the managers are working with the same goals, which should be to help people, to help the community and to elevate the level of care for its patients, when possible.

Another thing that we need to look at is to create a volunteer or a community support room for public education or basic training. Ideally, we could provide first aid, CPR, drug awareness courses, public safety courses and others to help instruct our co-responders, such as our local volunteer firefighters or first responders.

The final area to address is the availability of a meditation area or chapel. Someplace where you could go to debrief after a call or share your experiences in privacy and away from the public. Many of our informal debriefings are done over a coffee, after we have cleaned and restocked the units. The training room could still be used for bigger debriefings, which the public could also have access to.

Chapter 4: Changing the Bad – Fighting Negative Attitudes Head-on

"Fighting Negative Attitudes Head-on"

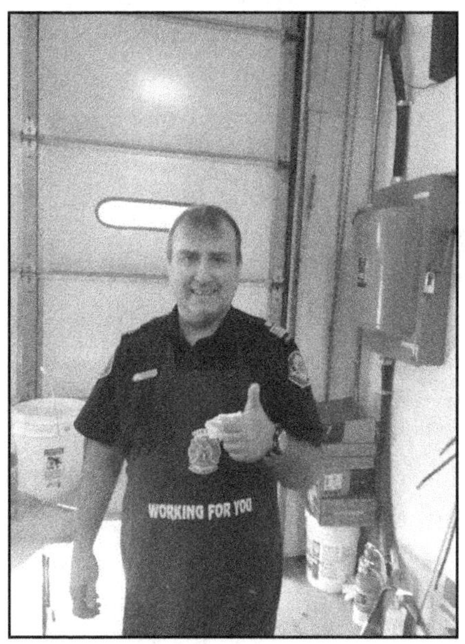

Know that it takes just one man to make a difference in others' lives. My friend Kevin is one of those people.

One thing that can destroy the EMS world is the promotion of the wrong attitude. When you start down the slippery slope of having a bad attitude, it only gets worse over time. Failures can be turned into success stories with the right person with the right attitude. You can take a small-town farm kid or a city kid and make their dreams a reality as long as they start down the right road from the very start. Both might have always wanted to be a paramedic, a firefighter or a police officer since they were old enough to crawl. It's funny how one simple toy or one kind act from one person can provide inspiration and change the destiny of everyone they touch.

I never dreamed of being a paramedic until one fateful day when one of my friends needed help and it never came. Jamie is the reason I have made it this far. I wonder how many EMS practitioners get into this profession for very similar reasons, or possibly to fill some hidden desire to make the world better off than before they came along. I look at my closest friends in EMS and in health care and they have similar attributes. They are often compassionate leaders, and they provide endless caring. They are dedicated to helping others for what are often deeply personal reasons.

The most gifted of my friends are the doctors, physicians and surgeons who get the last chance to intervene with very sick trauma patients. They work as a team, as a group that sticks together. Over the years they have mastered the art of mentoring those who follow in their footsteps. We need to somehow get to that level of mastering our team concepts, then somehow, some way, we will become a better profession.

We can take that same mentorship mentality and apply it to our team. We can mentor our EMS family to be a more unified body of practitioners. They, in turn, can work together and become a team that is unstoppable. You can take two completely different people, put them together and they can save a life using their collective knowledge. By promoting our profession, along with gifted leadership and a unified team approach, anything is possible. A team that is willing to learn and adapt to a changing environment will evolve and will make our profession sustainable.

The more we learn, the more we can intervene to help others survive impossible odds after sustaining tragedy or being in a medical disaster. One day, we will become a profession where there are no basic life support (BLS) or advanced life support (ALS) units, only the initial "Emergency Medicine" that responds, evaluates and initiates life-saving measures as they transport a patient to the appropriate facility. We need to be an extension of the health care team, all the way from the onset of the acute illness, monitoring the patient's progress until they are admitted to hospital and possibly when they are discharged, and then as community paramedics helping with home care assessments, treatments and referrals, to possibly end-of-life assistance for terminal patients.

In this world, if you want to survive, you must learn how to defeat any obstacle that you will face. In the 2017 movie *Wind River*, character Cory Lambert says it all too well: "Out here you survive, or you surrender." Our obstacles in the EMS world are unique but are not that different from those of other health care professions. Our environment is unique, and our resources are limited. Our level of diagnostic investigation is also limited, but we use our experience and intuition to undo decisions that we can live with. We make the best of bad situations and we look for solutions that are beneficial to our patients, their families and our crews. The EMS profession can create some great leaders as they progress from emergency medical responder to critical care paramedic status. Only by choosing to become a leader can you learn to defeat the negative world around you and thus impact the future.

Most people don't realize the influence that negative thoughts have. I will share with you a little secret. We all have been taught about the "fight or flight" instinct that is supported or stimulated by our sympathetic nervous system. It is amazing to learn that we can fight negative thoughts just as easily by thinking positive thoughts which directly activate the parasympathetic nervous system and help to calm us down. As paramedics and EMS providers, we constantly battle tragedy and chaos by taking charge of any situation and managing the scene. By using our visual input from our environment, we learn how to adapt and intervene in the most logical, most correct, order, depending on our patient's needs, and we complete these interventions in a timely manner.

The next time you go for a walk, I want you to look past your normal field of vision. Look toward the sky and take it all in: the sounds, the smells and how much the world has to offer. Many people take life for granted. It's not always going to be such a good day for others, and we see that all too often. If you just look beyond your normal circle of events you will help yourself in ways most don't or can't comprehend. I promise it will help you focus on positive change. It takes effort to drive away negative thoughts, but as they arise, visualize putting them on a shelf for a future time when you can ponder them and delete them from your normal thought patterns for good. Don't let evil win; drive it away with the goodness of the great things in our lives.

Our job requires us to use our primary senses of sight, sound, smell and touch to evaluate specific patient conditions. All the facts are immediately sent to our brain and solutions to our sensory input are instantly made. Many people take our primary sense of balance and our vestibular sense—our sense of position—for granted, but they keep us safe even when we are in critical situations and they are controlled so quickly we don't even know they are happening.

Next time you watch a crew doing an extrication from a motor vehicle crash, watch the motions and the reactions to the situations. You will be impressed at how flexible we can be and how strong we are in times of need. We can, and do, perform superhuman feats from time to time. I've had a 55 kg, or 115-lb. partner help me lift a 159 kg, or a 350-lb. person up out of a ditch on a spine board or a scoop more than once. This is while walking up a steep slope, trying to balance ourselves and, often, a non-cooperative patient. All the while, we are planning our next treatment options, talking to the co-rescuers and ignoring or blocking out the negative or vulgar language from the people we are trying to help. The pure strength and determination that is needed often comes from the heart of the rescuer.

With our ability to master our sense of balance and our vestibular sense, we have an increased ability to multitask at an even faster rate. Often, we see a gifted professional start a difficult intravenous line or insert an advanced airway. If you stop to think about it, anyone who excels at their art must have skill, dexterity, muscle memory, repeated practice, increased proficiency and a positive attitude to make what they do look so easy. We are the masters of our minds; we must allow our minds to grow constantly by interacting with the world around us. Only by taking over our thoughts and planning our actions do we learn how to master the hardest skills and increase our dexterity when it comes to physical and mental tasks. The art of running a code or being a trauma team leader is not something to be taken lightly; it takes years of experience and practice. The team is looking for our guidance to perform every skill, as well as to know when to implement it in the most logical timing. That's part of the art of mastering emergency medicine.

The first step to fighting a negative attitude is opening up one's senses. Your senses are much more powerful than most people suspect. Not only can they save your life in times of hazards, but they can also prevent us from entering a dangerous situation in the first place. Your view of the world needs to open peripherally. By using your peripheral vision, you're turning on or fine-tuning your situational awareness. Being aware of your surroundings is very influential when it comes to your ability to survive and see the good things in life. It also keeps you safe. While responding to EMS calls, we are always close to potential and actual hazards. Many of these hazards could easily harm or eliminate us if we are not careful. Some of these hazards are natural, unsafe environments and some are man-made, such as toxic gas, potential explosions, active shooters or other bad people that can make our day terrible.

By using your peripheral vision, you become more aware of your environment and can learn to come up with solutions to complications as they arise. It's like always having a flexible backup plan without ever needing to use it. But you have it just the same.

A positive outlook helps you become a better EMS professional as well as ensuring that you are always assessing your situation or environment and noticing potential concerns or helpful tools. You can never be too careful. Partners should always be watching out for each other 24/7, 365 days a year.

Sometimes we get so focused on the task at hand that we miss seeing the rest of the real world. It's an instinct derived from needing to protect yourself with threats always around you. It's very often thought of as watching for potential enemies or trying to sneak through without anyone seeing you. You're always a target or someone is always hunting you like prey. If you're so focused on hazards or potential hazards, you risk missing the good things around us. We need a happy medium of looking out for harm as well as looking for the beautiful or nurturing environmental aspects that enlighten our day.

The one sense that many people take for granted is the ability to hear. Our hearing often protects us from unseen dangers. If you're working in a violent area, you expect some degree of danger, as opposed to being on a transfer unit, where the days are mostly uneventful. Other than the odd medical emergency, you will be completely unscathed at the end of your shift. The sounds of silence and the warning sounds of impending danger are never to be taken for granted.

We should not take for granted the sound of music nor the sound of silence. To find positive music that opens your awareness is so fulfilling. Imagine the moment when you are sitting in front of a great performer and feeling the music in your heart and enriching your soul. That's the feeling and therapeutic emotion you need to drive out the bad days. That same emotion can also help you to help others. Music therapy has been around for years and it can be very beneficial for sick and injured people in the right context. At the opposite end of the spectrum lies the sound of silence; it can be scary if you're auscultating a chest in a small child, yet it can be peaceful after a long, hard day.

All our senses are unique and every one of us has slightly different abilities which make us more adaptive to certain situations. To be able to sit and hold someone's hand as they share their life events with you is priceless. To anticipate or relate to others' needs and feelings is also an art. It's most commonly referred to as the "art of caring." It's the one part you can't teach, and it can't be passed on from a book. Not everyone can master it. Some can do it on their very first call but later, after you're tired, it can be harder to give out for obvious reasons. You can only give so much before you need to recharge or have some time off and recharge your body and soul, so that you can keep functioning at an optimal level.

The starting point to fixing negative attitudes is at the student level. I would set the tone for my classes on the first day and in the first few minutes of every class, I would stress that EMS is not about someone excelling on one's own. This profession is about teamwork, being accountable for our actions, being willing to learn, being able to accept constructive feedback and mostly being able to evolve to the next level of prehospital provider. We all need to start someplace and part of being the new person, is that you must to be able to master the art of being an active listener, being someone that your partner wants to work beside on a ninety-six-hour tour. There is nothing worse than coming to work and, when it's time to go on a call, your partner starts complaining about the nature of the call they are being dispatched to. That can end one's professional career in a hurry. In this occupation, you need to enjoy performing the basics of care or you're not going to be of much use to anyone, least of all your patients.

One thing everyone needs to remember is that students and practitioners are the same in many aspects. Most people assume certain traits when they are in uniform. Although they function at different levels of care, a new paramedic can be saved by a primary care medic

(PCP) many times, especially at the start of their career. Likewise, a good EMR will help save lives long before the BLS or ALS arrive on scene. I may never understand why certain people are born to lead, and others are meant to follow, but that is the world we work in and live in. We need to be able to adapt to everyone we work with. Not everyone we work with will be born leaders, but if you're in a helping profession it's for a reason. The reasons are many, but at the end of the day we are all in it for the people.

We often walk into a busy emergency room or onto a ward and feel the negativity there hanging in the air like a looming storm. Then, the next busy emergency, the doctors and nurses are bending over backwards to help us in any way they can. I know that one bad apple can spoil a whole batch of apples, so the lesson of the day is "Do not be the bad apple." Be the first one to cheer up your group every day. Be the one who never lets his or her coworkers down. When you next walk into a busy ER and see a smile coming your way, you have found a good person. A good person that can make your day better and, ultimately, improve your patient's day as well.

Often with the right attitude, by displaying caring and compassion, you can change the forecast and make the sun shine down on everyone. That is when the real patient care is initiated. It's hard to report to a nurse who is not interested in your patient, especially in front of the family. The only way to move forward is with kindness. If you can connect with one person in the receiving hospital, then you have someone on your team. That is how teams are built, and the more people on your team, the more success stories you can create together.

Having the right team members means simply having the good ones on your side.

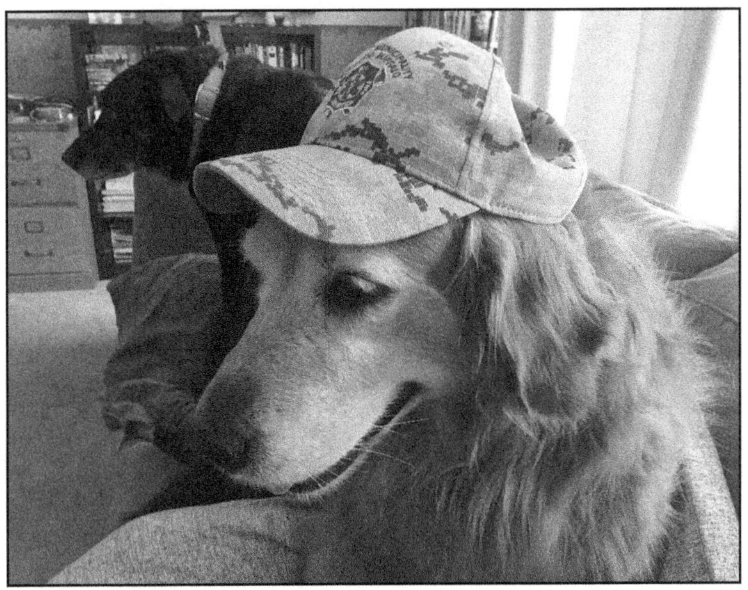

Pebbles and Ember – part of a winning team

Chapter 5: Finding the Right Team Members

"To make the right team, you need the right people from the very start to be successful."

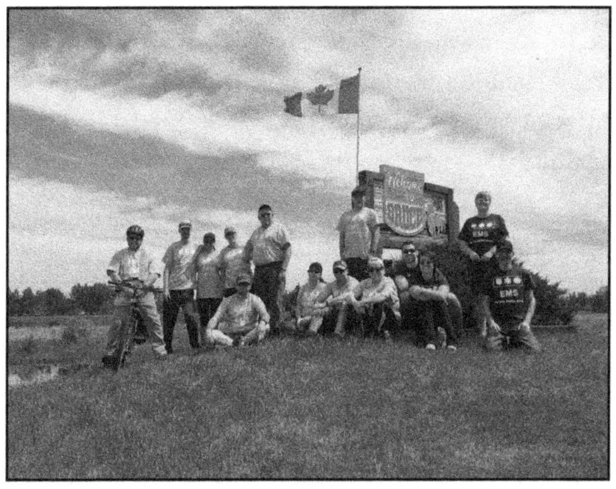

#NoOneWalksAlone2017: Dale's team

When building a Dream Team, you need staff who want to be part of it. The EMS system would work perfectly with a basic life support (BLS) and advanced life support (ALS) model as a primary emergency response system. We could use a primary care paramedic (PCP) and an advanced care paramedic (ACP) on every unit, as well as add staff when the situation was more complex, or the acuity was noted to be high. On those calls we could even add an emergency medical responder (EMR) and a critical care paramedic (CCP) from time to time. When I think about all the people I know who have been excellent staff members, I realize they had some things in common:

1) they all liked animals or pets;
2) they liked to work as a team; and
3) they were willing to put in the extra time to excel.

Many dedicated staff even came in after-hours to attend study sessions to make up for the perceived gaps in the current education modules. The most important commonality was they wanted to help people, so they easily fit in to our service.

If we had extra staff for training and extra units providing care, we could provide an enhanced level of care for our community members. We could run a transfer unit, as well, staffed with BLS or ALS workers. With supervisors in rapid response units or paramedic response units (PRU), we would have it made. All we had to do was get the right staff and pair them up with the right partner, and team building would happen on its own. My thoughts turned to my last couple of primary care paramedic classes and of those students' strengths and weaknesses. Every class was uniquely different and certain students excelled for many reasons.

Team members would need to be assigned together in a way that blended their strengths and that lessened the impact of their individual weaknesses. The team would always be enhanced if just the right two people were together. You need one person with Type-A personality traits, as they tend to not procrastinate and are better at time management. They make decisions and live with the results. They plan out calls and can organize the day to make it more logical. Some Type-As say they have trouble understanding the perceived stupidity of others, but that's just a minor flaw. They also can have trouble with the concept of not being able to do something on every call to help every patient in need. If something can be physically done, they are always willing to try it, if it could possibly help a patient. Their mind will always find a logical solution to any given situation.

After some research, I was enlightened that Type-A people are most likely and most willing to learn something from a call after it is completed. A retrospective review of the call and the outcomes is very helpful to them in the learning process. Type-A people are generally very active and view laziness as a character flaw and wouldn't be caught dead sitting around and watching the world go past.

It has been said that Type-A people are more passionate in their patient care and will go the extra mile to make a difference in the outcomes. I feel this usually applies to me, but I can also shut it off some days and be "Type Z," which means that I don't care at all. When I do something, it's got to be meaningful and for an ethical or logical reason. Even if I must bend the rules to save a life, I will do it. The only drawback is that I can be too passionate, and because we are often set up for defeat due to the terrible situations we face, it can make post-call processing difficult and painful. It can be hard on our psyche and we can be discouraged after having several bad outcomes in a row, as we take it personally. This can ultimately make us more likely to suffer from PTSD or compassion fatigue. When I think about my past bad calls, I consider how therapy would have helped me. I thought some more and tried to come up with ways to predict work-related complications.

My solution was to watch the crew's responses to extra-stressful calls, and potentially taking them off-car or out of service for a few hours after a harder call to let them regroup. Some crew members have kids and stressful home lives, and many have seen prior stressful events and it is imperative to get feedback from your co-workers during every call. You need to know their weaknesses and strengths as well as your own. Often, as a call progressed, I could see the changes in my partner's demeanor due to the type of call we were on. We all have our breaking points and we are all just human. No matter your level of expertise, you can reach a saturation point when dealing with the lives of others and their problems.

I always liked to be partnered with someone with some obsessive-compulsive (OCD) traits. These people have an increased number of unwanted and repetitive thoughts, feelings, ideas, sensations or obsessions about getting something right every time. Their personal behaviours drive them to do something over and over again until they get it perfect. This can come in handy when ensuring units are always checked, stocked, and properly cleaned, and people with these OCD tendencies can be counted on to do the same thing every time, even when they are exhausted. I thought about some of my past partners and realized how they helped keep me out of harm's way even when I didn't realize it. There is no magical formula for the right partner, but when you have a winning team any difficulty can be overcome if it is humanly possible.

My winning team was a gift sent from heaven. The day shift was uneventful, and I was very grateful to be partnered with Julie. I had great respect for her as she would always make sure we had a good day no matter what. We would face it together. Connor was our other partner and was just there to make sure I stayed out of trouble. Sometimes I think destiny was on my side even when hell was opposing us. We were called to a motor vehicle crash at an open intersection. Dispatch said there were two patients and one serious. Our co-responders (the fire department, the police and additional units) were already deployed. Julie had her strengths and Connor had his unique personality. They had my back and I had theirs. In theory we had nothing to worry about. Well, so I thought. I was soon to realize I was dead wrong.

On arrival, we parked so that we could protect our side of the accident by using our unit as a shield. This was so we could protect ourselves from other drivers on the roadway. It never surprised me how many people would try to drive through an accident site and not care about our safety. I've been almost hit twice, but thankfully others kept me safe both times. Julie took the trauma kit and Connor grabbed the ALS airway bag. I brought up the rear and tried to get a good overview of the scene. They both knew what had to be done without any direction from me.

As we approached, we could smell the strong odor of gasoline. There were no visible flames. There was no sign of fire, but I realized the hair was standing up on the back of my neck. That meant a ruptured fuel tank. I looked back, and the first responding fire trucks were about half a kilometre away still. I said, "Let's triage. Keep your heads up," to my partners and they smiled back and acknowledged me with a head nod as they split up to each take one of the vehicles involved. We all went to work knowing that we were already in imminent danger.

There are some sounds you can never forget. Some sounds are good sounds, and some are bad sounds. The next sound I heard was not what we needed or wanted to hear, but it was there just the same: the distinct crackling sound of fire. I could not see it, but I knew what it was right away. Julie had just reached the driver of the small blue Honda Civic. Her patient looked to be alive and awake. That's always a good sign in any big trauma call. Connor's patient didn't look as good. The Honda had nailed the driver's door, and that is devastating for any driver at any time. I was praying we could perform self-extrication if it was at all possible. We had a few seconds to decide and our success would depend on just a little more than luck today. If we made the wrong decision, we could lose both our patients and possibly our own lives. If we waited for the responding fire trucks, we increased the chances of losing two more lives. Only time and a small miracle would make this outcome more positive. It's never too late to say a prayer for everyone involved.

Connor was just reaching for a pulse through the driver's side window of the Ford F-350 truck. Then I could see the problem as flames suddenly erupted from the Honda. I looked and saw a fuel tank in the truck on its side in the back. In split second, I made my mind up and I yelled to them both as I radioed our mayday to the responding units. We could simply back out and wait for the fire staff to clear the hazards, but if we did that we could potentially lose lives. If we stayed, we could all be vaporized. I said, "Extract them or we all need to leave." Whatever we did, it would be as a team. Those were the only options we had left. We had run out of all other options. Our survival skills were being put to the test. It was the perfect time to *run* just like Forest Gump from the famous movie of the same name.

We all knew it was now or never. As I came up behind Connor, he yelled, "He's unconscious, but alive." Julie simultaneously pulled open the door of the Honda and grabbed the female driver. In a second, she was doing a fireman's carry and they were off. God, she could run like the wind even with a woman across her shoulders. Now I just needed to convince Connor to get the heck out of the danger zone. Then he grinned at me, and I knew without his saying a word that that grin meant "It's a good day to die." He knew the hazards and he knew the risk.

Time slowed down for me as I computed the egress options and hazards and calculated the time we had left. Somewhere in the back of my mind I heard the old saying that it's "better to be dead and cool, then alive and uncool." But that didn't say anything about being toasted alive or burned to death. Burning to death was not the way I wanted to go. And it was not the way my co-workers should have to go as well. For sure it was not the way for our patients die.

I went to Connor and said, "It's now or never, my friend," to which he replied, "I'm not leaving without him." I shook my head. I knew he would say that, and I also knew we had one chance and that was it. We both grabbed hold of the door and we pulled as hard as we could. In a fraction of a second, the door popped open. Who needs the Jaws of Life when you have two very strong EMS staff jacked up on adrenalin and Timmy's coffee? Connor reached for the patient and I grabbed my folding EMS knife and cut the seat belt in one slice. No matter the internal injuries, we had to leave. Connor was getting resistance from the patient's trapped legs. I reached in and cleared his legs from the brake pedal. They were broken but attached. I yelled "Go!" In the next moment we were free; Connor had the patient and was off. I grabbed the ALS airway bag, and as I reached for the trauma bag beside the Honda, the fire started to bloom. I thought I could get it, but it might not be worth dying for and this was way past being serious. I knew the kit was expensive, but decided it was replaceable and left it. Today, it was an acceptable loss.

We could get another trauma bag. As we ran, the fire became human and the sound of death was immediately behind us. I knew we were too close, but I also knew we had someone on our side who would look after us all. Someday, your faith will count for everything. I also knew if it was my day to die saving a life, it was okay with me if my partners made it away safe. I could be the sacrifice if one was needed. The Honda erupted into flames, which then leapt to the truck to burn. I knew we were still alive, so we had a fighting chance. Time was against us, though. The noise of a raging fire is something you never forget.

Julie had dropped her patient off on the far side of the unit and was running at us as fast as she could when the fuel tank from the truck exploded directly behind us. We all went down in a big pile of people, but thankfully we were all okay. We were far enough away not to get burned. We had defeated the angel of death today. We quickly checked each other out for injuries and grabbed our patient and the ALS airway kit and headed to the unit. A police officer had the back door open and a stretcher was coming out as we approached. The second unit, as well as the fire crews, were now on scene. The cavalry was here. We were lucky; even if the patient was injured, at least he was still alive.

Several hours later, it finally hit us that we almost got vaporized. My personal protection vest had a fragment of metal lodged in it, proving it was also stab-proof. I'm sure we had a guardian angel on our side that day. We don't normally expect to run while on an EMS call, but today we'd had no other option.

The fire crews took over as we retreated to safety. They immediately set up an attack line to cool the flames. They let us get our patients loaded and then we backed out to a safer zone. The second unit came in and grabbed the second patient and then backed up to a safe zone as well. The fire crews were then able to withdraw to a safer zone, and we heard the final boom as the tank in the back of the truck erupted and sent pieces of metal and flames shooting skyward. We had lost our trauma bag for good, but it was the only casualty of the entire event. A supervisor from the PRU then pulled up and jumped into our unit. I told him we lost a trauma bag but that was it. He quickly radioed and got the third responding unit to come to our aid with an extra trauma kit. They also helped with patient care until we could hear again. We all had been too close to the explosion and had temporarily lost our hearing. That was my third time in my career that I'd been so close to an explosion, so I knew I was stretching my luck. I would not get a fourth time.

Our supervisor took over the patient care along with the BLS crew. We were delegated to participating bystanders. In no time, we were headed toward the trauma centre and everyone on board was given a task, be it starting IVs, getting airway equipment ready, preparing medications or applying the ALS principles of critical care. The additional police and fire staff followed with the extra unit and the supervisor's vehicle. The other ALS unit followed the convoy of emergency vehicles carrying the patient from the Honda who was only slightly injured. They also had an extra staff member driving for them, so they could tag team for any patient care that needed to be done. There was much to be done, but everyone had a role, and in no time, patient care was organized and initiated. An extra firefighter could retrieve the PRU when they were free, after the fire scene was secured.

On that day, not only was our initial patient assessment interrupted, but all our initial treatments were, too. The call was not managed "textbook style," but more like a military or a hostage recovery attempt. Julie had her patient and Connor had his. I had them all accounted for, so I was ready to declare it a successful mission regardless of the outcomes for our patients. They both gave me the thumbs-up sign as we departed the scene. I smiled back with a few tears in my eyes, knowing all too well how close we came to losing it all today. I would go to hell and back for my partners and today showed me they would do the same for me, as well. They had just proved to themselves that they were made for this profession. I was a little upset that I had let them get into danger when I knew better. It was something we did even if we shouldn't, but it was who we were.

On this call, we didn't even get a chance to perform simple airway manoeuvres or to stop any bleeding; it was not possible. On the initial approach, we had a patient and we knew there were hazards, but it wasn't until we were already in the hot zone that we realized we were in serious trouble. But our patients were counting on us. It was then that I realized that, no matter how well you screened people, you didn't know how they would act or respond until the pressures were at their highest. When the right people gathered together, they somehow created a synergistic effect. There was not a better team than all the people involved that day, from the police officers to the firefighters and the EMS staff.

With just the right partners on our team, we can save lives, and we can change outcomes despite the challenges or the personal dangers we come across. The hurdles that come with working in our profession are not always visible but are the consequences of situations. It just proved my hypothesis that things happen for a reason. Today we had an extra staff member due to a scheduling mishap and it turned out to work in our favour. Two people on this response would have been the norm, but today had not been a normal day. Today fate and destiny made the impossible happen for a reason. When we needed three people to perform a life-saving miracle, they were there.

It seemed I had lost track of time. That was when I realized the blast had been just a little too close for comfort. I had likely sustained a little more of the blast and was the oldest on scene. I also had a history of concussions. The signs of concussion are usually evident, but often it's others around you who see them first. The first time I realized there was something wrong was when we were pulling into the trauma hospital and the trauma team took over from us.

It was then that my partners realized that the last hour was a complete blur for me. I wasn't sure how things got done, and I realized that I had likely suffered a concussion, either because of the explosion, or from hitting the ground afterwards a little too hard. It was then that we got to hold each other and say thank you to our fellow team members. We all shed some tears of joy but also had to shake off the fear. I took one look at Julie and said, "You're nominated for the hundred-yard relay from now on." I then said to Connor, "And you are my pick for the new tactical medic position." They both smiled and gave me long, hard hug. I said to them both quietly, so no one else could hear, "That was just too close, my friends," which was too close even if they were both angels and for that I was sorry.

We slowly got our group together and piled into the units to head back to the base. On the way home, we did our own debriefing in the back of the unit. We were out of service and our shift was being extended even if we were not going back to work. We all knew today was one of those days that we would never forget. Nothing short of a miracle kept us safe that day. I had seen close calls before but that was too close for anyone.

I thought long and hard about the call and I wondered what the odds were that Julie had attended to the woman who was easily extricated. Our extraction had been more difficult and we both needed to be in the right place of time to make it work. If we had been five to ten seconds slower, it would have been game over for all of us. But a minute sooner, and two people would have died a terrible death. Nothing can change our destiny if we sit back and wait for the outcomes to be decided. Some days, we are forced to take chances and we know the risk, even if we don't really think about it carefully or add up the odds against us. Today we made the right decisions and time was on our side, but only just.

On the way home, I fell asleep, only to be awoken by my crew as we arrived at the base. I hadn't been easy to rouse, so I got a visit to the local ER with a worried set of partners, and the local ER staff got me triaged, in no time, I was seen, assessed and a CT scan was done. Somehow my brain had survived a lifetime of being banged up and was still structurally intact. I could officially add one more concussion to the list. I was put off work for a week and told "No lifting or EMS duties." Anyone who knows me knows that I'm not much of a person to complain but I knew my brain needed a rest, so I heeded their instructions. A damaged brain always wants you to sleep and let time and rest heal it. I slept a little more as the nurses kept an eye on me.

I was picked up by my co-workers and taken home. I had no plans but to sleep, but they insisted on staying over and made themselves at home with my dogs. They took them for a quick run behind the local Walmart. I put my comfy clothes on and immediately fell asleep on the couch. It was not a good night. The nightmare started sometime after I hit REM sleep. I woke up in fear. I could see and hear the flames; I could feel heat. Anyone who has seen bad accidents knows the one fear we all have: fire. I had no desire to burn to death. I would settle for falling off my deck and breaking my neck any day. That would be a less evil way to go. Burning to death or watching people burn to death is not something we first responders ever want to talk about.

I had no idea how long I was asleep, but when I woke up, both my partners were at my side. They stayed and made sure I would be okay. They had not even gone to sleep. They were just hanging out with my puppies and they knew I needed them even if I had no clue they were there. They made themselves at home and put on music and ensured the puppies and cats were spoiled rotten.

After I woke up, I shared some of my past call stories. The burned patients to the very bad crashes. The sounds and the sensory input from the smells never gets forgotten. As soon as I heard the sound of the flames yesterday, I had known we were in trouble, but it was not something we could ever turn away from. My co-worker had also known we were in trouble, but we stood our ground as a team. It was one time in the space-time continuum we could challenge the outcomes for two unsuspecting souls. I apologized for letting them take the risk even when I knew we should not have entered an unsafe zone. They replied that we didn't have a choice. It was an acceptable risk.

Over time, we all shared stories and we shared our fears and our happy memories, as well. I got to know more about them, and I shared with them stuff that I had not shared with anyone else. It was a time when I felt completely safe to share anything. Most times, the bonds created over blood, sweat and tears are stronger than any other friendships.

We were now family. An EMS family is not a blood family, but the bonds are earned, and after we performed together in a very stressful event, our bonds were for life. Nothing could ever take our wins or loses away from us. We earned them and paid for them in sweat and blood. We shared the pain and we shared the joy of every successful outcome. Sharing both pain and joy is part of being a team.

After breakfast, I felt better, but I also was beyond tired, so it was time to sleep some more. A sleeping pill and two extra-strength Tylenol for the headache, and I was out. Many hours later I woke up from a very relaxing dream. It allowed me to come to terms with the events from the past day. I had even settled some old battles. The act of sharing our bad days lessens the load and helps us deal with the future.

My partners had headed home after breakfast and they were sleeping now, I was sure. My headache was gone but the rest of me felt like I just fought with Rocky. I then realized I was surrounded by my pets. There were my puppies and Socks, the cat, who thought he was a golden retriever. I never got around to telling him he was conflicted. Fuzzy was sleeping at my feet and purring so loud. I was thinking about the events of the last twenty-four hours. I thought about my partners and what they meant to me and how special they both were. They were angels both in and out of uniform.

I could never thank them enough for the extra care they provided me. God, we came so close to being in big trouble. It was the calls like that made us become a team. I then thought about it some more and realized that they were also bonding as friends. We all shared the worst of our fears without ever feeling like we were at fault or we had done wrong, even if we shared some of the blame. My next shifts would be so rewarding, even if I knew I needed to slowly walk away from it all as soon as Sarah was ready to assume my role. The last two days made me think of many things. I was listening to a song and somehow it rang true to me today. Sometimes we can't always be the strong one. Some days we need others to help us when we are done. The song "Just be Held" by Casting Crowns had a message that resonated with my soul. It can be a message to all of us if you just listen and let it touch your heart.

Hold it together
Everyone needs you strong
But life hits you out of nowhere
And barely leaves you holding on.

And when you're tired of fighting
Chained by your control
There's freedom in surrender
Lay it down and let it go

So, when you're on your knees and
Answers seem so far away
You're not alone, stop holding on and just be held
Your world's not falling apart, it's falling into place
I'm on the throne, stop holding on and just be held
Just be held, just be held.

I don't think you have to be religious or have a specific belief to care about others. If you share your life to help people in times of need, you will see times when your battles are great, and your successful outcomes dwindle away. We simply take what is given to us and make the best out of it. We are entitled to have bad days. We are entitled to have times where we need to let down our defences. We can't always be strong and the ones who are immune to tears. Even Superman cries sometimes.

When we are with the right people they will protect us and, no matter what we face, they will have our backs. No matter how big or terrible the tragedies we face we should know at the end of the day we are never alone. We can't always be the leader and sometimes we must entrust our co-workers to watch our backs when we need a break. That's what our EMS teams need to work on in the future. We need to share our wins and our losses to better understand how to cope with the battles we face both physically, mentally and spiritually. We need to make our profession a closer-knit team.

Over the years, we receive more help then we give.

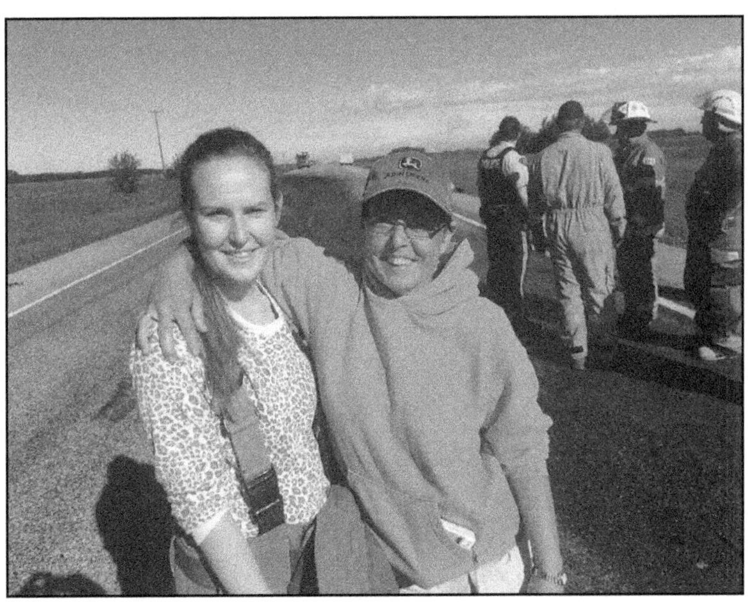

My EMS family has my back 24/7 – and I have theirs…

Chapter 6: Setting Up the Perfect Response System

"Providing Proper Care"

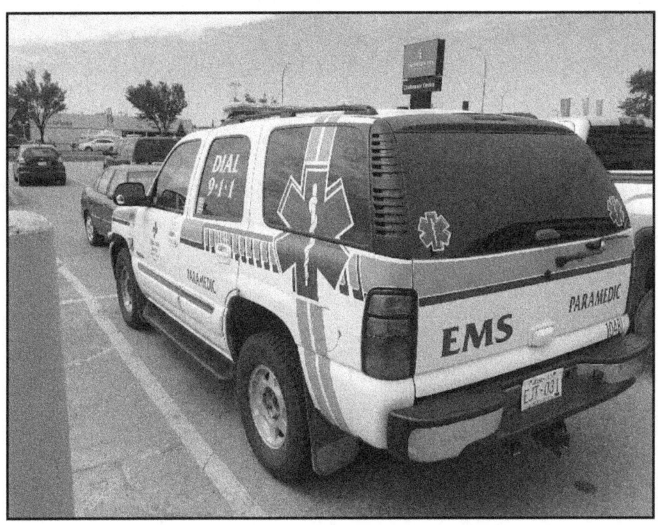

Paramedic response unit (PRU) vs. EMS backup

The history of using only an ambulance for EMS response and how we respond to calls has transformed in the last ten years. Over the last decade, we have developed response vehicles with specialized equipment. While present and easily recognizable in urban centres, an appropriate incarnation of the PRU continues to evolve in rural areas. Often, we don't need another ambulance on scene, as there's usually only one patient to care for, but an extra set of hands or rapid access to an individual with extra experience is often required. The birth and development of paramedic response units (PRUs) is one of the most streamlined ways to provide quick, efficient, advanced care by paramedics in our urban communities.

Decades ago, when the norm of routine calls was only a few per day, regular ambulances with BLS capabilities sufficed. But those days are long gone. Saving lives has elevated to an art form based on modern science, and when practiced properly, makes the difference for people in need. The proper practice of advanced life support (ALS) offers many more options for sick and injured patients. While a "higher level" of health care is now more uniform, there remains a long way to go for the present standards to be considered the benchmark in care.

It is now possible for paramedics to perform advanced skills on scene or on the side of the road, interventions that were traditionally only done in an active emergency room. For example, we can now inject clot-busting medication for an acute heart attack on-scene, and this relatively minor intervention has radically changed the outcomes for acute heart-attack patients. Another recent advancement in care for suspected cerebral vascular emergencies is to bring a mobile CT scanner in the back of an ambulance and meet EMS crews on the side of the road or in rural locations upon request and through online medical control. The future of the EMS world is being challenged, adapted and enhanced by the level of care we are now offering to our patients.

As well, we have started working in critical care areas of busy hospitals and are active as community paramedics in providing end-of-life care for palliative patients. We have literally gone from a "scoop-and-run" service twenty years ago to now caring for acute and chronically ill patients in their own home environments. Community medicine continues to evolve as a field, thanks in part to increased public education. We need to continue to be active in the role of public education to ensure that preventative strategies become common knowledge for the layperson. An obvious and easy way to help the younger generation is for them to become better educated and better trained in standard first aid, along with learning how to perform CPR. Moreover, it would not be difficult to add elementary competence of Emergency Medical Responder

(EMR) coursework for high school students, perhaps as part of their career and life management studies.

As the population increases, call volumes increase, and complexity also increases proportionately. Over the last several years, we have become more than just ambulance drivers and our scope of practice needs to exceed beyond that of traditional providers. We have incorporated new ideas such as a paramedic response unit (PRU). This idea has flexed from having a higher level of care on-site, such as a physician or paramedic, to just a paramedic in some regions. Ideally, the higher the available level of care, coupled with a decreased response time, the more lives that can be saved. Some countries such as England run an emergency physician in a fast response vehicle, so in some ways, we are still behind the trends.

With the use of a flexible PRU, we can respond more quickly within a community. The addition of PRU vehicles obviously increases the number of response vehicles and can statistically provide on-scene ALS care even in times of ambulance shortages, such as when ambulances need to clean up and restock from a previous call before coming on scene. As public levels of basic first aid knowledge increase, it is not unusual to see paramedics being assisted by volunteers, or to have first responders perform life-saving manoeuvres prior to an ambulance arriving. Then, after the patient is treated or stabilized, they can assist the crews with the transport of the patients to the most appropriate hospital. The crew can then assume patient care and the PRU is able to return to service immediately if needed. The PRUs are often utilized when ambulances are not available, which can be a little unnerving for the single paramedic.

Patient needs have dictated that extra equipment be added and that staffing levels be increased in proportion to the demographics of a particular area. If only we could drop off our patients in an urban hospital and leave; those days are long gone. It's not uncommon to see six to ten EMS units at a city hospital waiting for the next available bed in a backlogged system. It's very hard to justify adding extra ambulances to an already stressed system, when a PRU could be added at about half the cost, only one staff instead of two making it a great cost-saving measure.

On simple "treat-and-release" calls, one can completely forgo an ambulance, especially as a PRU can be on scene, perform a quick triage and arrange the most appropriate resources long before a unit ever becomes available. Every community is unique, and the calls will be unique to the population base we serve. As communities grow and the health care industry evolves, response numbers will increase. The number of emergency calls and the corresponding transfers will also increase over time.

Staffing requirements need to be tailored to the type of emergencies to which they typically respond in order to be effective or to improve the quality of patient care. In an ideal world, each patient would be attended to in less than ten minutes with either a basic life support (BLS) or an advanced life support (ALS) unit, but this is very cost-prohibitive. One urban compromise is to have the local firefighters (or other first responders) attend to reduce the time that it takes for patients to be attended to. It might work in an urban location to have an EMS provider at your side in less than ten minutes, but in rural and remote locations, it is usually not possible.

Response time in rural/remote locations can range from forty-five to sixty minutes, if everything falls into place. Some areas are lucky enough to have a medical response from a local volunteer fire department or by local first responders. This is a very good option for more remote locations that is both practical and life-saving. It's hard to achieve ALS care in all locations when our current system is not willing to even provide a good BLS service.

Ideally, a BLS unit would be dispatched initially, with an ALS unit standing by as potential backup. When those needs were not met in urban settings, the notion of a paramedic in a rapid response vehicle backed up by an ambulance arriving shortly thereafter to transport the patient become an economical solution. With extensive cooperation by volunteer firefighters, or rural first responders, along with other responding agencies coupled with some advanced planning and practice, most people can have equal access to emergency care when it's needed.

The biggest debate is: What is the "optimal" level of care? What I'm proposing is not a difficult concept to grasp. The educational systems, structural and logistical framework already exist. If there are doctors everywhere, and nurses everywhere, why can't there also be paramedics everywhere? I would suggest they are essential practitioners. The days of communities and cities going without paramedics should be in the past; as a profession we won't survive if we are too short-sighted about our future needs. If we don't educate ourselves, promote ourselves and increase our scope of practice, we are selling our profession short.

We need to be at the top of our game to service a complex and challenging world. Having a PRU or an extra unit available to respond to a baby in distress, a sudden arrest at a local school or an extra set of hands at a motor vehicle crash is worth it to help save a life. Any life saved would offset the cost of the essential services the PRU staff could provide. In many emergency situations, time is against us from the second the tragedy strikes. Once a patient's heart rate or breathing becomes ineffective, seconds matter. The nature of the emergency and the time it takes to arrive on scene almost always makes a difference in our ability to save a life. However, it must be acknowledged that, after a certain period, lives are lost no matter the intervention, such as when the heart is stopped for too long, or the patient goes into a state of irreversible shock.

A PRU is set up to be a rapid response 4X4 and is made for on or off-road capabilities. It stocks our complete BLS, airway, and ALS kits, as well as a LP-15 monitor, extra disaster equipment and supplemental oxygen. It also has extra blankets and an emergency patient moving belt (essentially a big blanket with handles). Moreover, it carries extra lighting, flares, radio batteries, a charger base and extra LP charger with two spare batteries. On board also are two emergency tactical stretchers, Narcan, triage tags and extra patient charts for use in the event of bigger disasters and mass casualty situations.

Combat-style tourniquets are now essential in every trauma kit; even the police are carrying them for their effectiveness in stopping extremity bleeding. They are simply called a CAT tourniquet.

Most PRUs are made to handle more like a large SUV than a three-ton truck. They are staffed by one senior paramedic, so they are a great asset to any emergency medical situation. In some urban centres, the PRUs are rapid response cars, but because they are not able to carry much extra equipment and have limited space for extra staff, these would not be as practical in rural locations.

Another idea is to simply ensure that local fire departments and fire medical co-responders are trained to sufficiently assess hazards and are adequately equipped. Many of our first responders are trained as fire medical responders or as emergency medical responders. Other provinces with similar needs have utilized local volunteers to cover most of the province, even in remote areas. Volunteers could certainly stand to receive more hands-on training with current EMS services. EMS can always use extra hands in day-to-day emergency situations; even offering extra training in driving the units would benefit everyone.

Ideally, it would be a routine practice to utilize the volunteers to keep their skills current and ensure they are always receiving continuing education. What better way than to have a fire medical responder (FMR) or an EMR on every call who could either lead or offer assistance with the calls (depending on their complexity). On an easy BLS call they could be in charge, and if it was a critical situation, the ALS or the critical care paramedics would take over and assume control.

Let's then take the current emergency medical responders (EMR) and make them either specialists in medical response or let them stay as FMRs. Currently, EMRs need additional training to bridge the gap in proper care. The first component is the driving module and the second is more advanced symptom relief or expanded medical therapeutic training. Education is not cheap, but the cost to train a limited number of responders would prove to be worth it in times of medical or traumatic emergencies that exceed local EMS responders' capabilities.

They must learn what the requirements are from our perspective as well to properly assume the role we all play in making the community safer, healthier, and accountable. Meeting with EMS members and becoming educated about our computer-aided dispatch system and call statistics, would help them to understand the system. It's easy to say that when there are no ambulances available to attend to a call, first responders can wait for fifteen to thirty minutes on neighbouring EMS services to attend. But when someone is bleeding out or their heart is stopped, the lost time is the biggest detriment to patient survival. We need to ensure that our co-responders have our backup when it is needed. They should not be expected to deal with the situation for a long period of time.

The first use of our new PRU did not go as expected. Our day started out very well as we were doing our best to keep our new Tahoe clean after a night of rain and the sun was now shining. Connor and I were on the new PRU doing training and making backup plans for the service. We were talking about staging and response criteria when we were called to assist a local sheriff at a rural motor vehicle collision (MVC). The local police were also dispatched, but we were the closest EMS vehicle. We took the most direct and safest route to get on scene in about ten minutes.

The local fire staff and multiple extra police were also being dispatched. The urgent code 10-33 suddenly came up, as the officer in question was now in immediate distress of some sort. It was unknown to us why. We were going to see how fast we could safely get on-scene without getting pulled over. We might get written up, but that was something for which we could ask for forgiveness later. It would not be our first time trying to do the impossible. The fastest way there was by air, but we needed to keep all our tires touching the ground.

We were hoping for more information as we drove toward the scene, but we knew that most likely it was a solo officer. I know from experience if you are actively defending yourself, you won't be able to talk or key your mic. The problems with rural responses are many: the distance is greater and the roads and traffic are unpredictable. There are no two days where the conditions are the same. Today we were on dry pavement and the traffic was sparse, which were both in our favour.

I was driving, and Connor was my spotter. We were making sure to arrive alive but also not to waste time getting to the scene. As we crested a hill, we could see the police cruiser parked behind and beside a rolled truck that was partly in the ditch. Connor said over the wailing sirens, "They're fighting with the officer," and I replied, "I'm going to come in hard and fast and lock it up." I quickly eyed my partner and I knew we were in a spot we were not supposed to be in. It was a tough spot, but it was part of the job. We could never delete the dangers or the hazards in our complex, unruly world. I said with confidence, "Are you ready?" Connor looked into my eyes and replied, "Hell, yeah!"

When I was almost on top of the scene, I locked up the PRU by pushing the brakes as hard as possible. We did a perfect skid and stopped parallel to the officer in trouble. She was actively fighting with two people and it looked like she was fighting for her life. Now was the time to forget staging and save a life if possible. Normally, we could stage but seeing as she was out numbered, it was our day to even up the score. They were about to find that we would do anything and everything to help our teammates. We were the worst two people to get backed into a corner and they would soon learn that the hard way.

Connor was out of the vehicle even before the vehicle was fully stopped and was running at maximum speed. He immediately did a flying tackle and took out a big man with what looked to be a piece of metal in his hand. I was out of the truck in a matter of seconds and I hit the other one as he turned toward me. I never saw the knife until later, but it didn't matter; I took him down with my first hit, then I was upon him. He was only dazed but, in seconds, I had him in a hold he could not break and then he was out. My tactics were not textbook, but they worked every time. There is only one rule when you fight for your life and that's to fight to win. But you win only by being the fastest, toughest, and by using just the right force. You don't second-guess what you need to do or you could already be dead. It comes down to "fight or flight," and today it was fight.

In mere seconds, Connor had his guy on the ground and pinned. I reached over to the officer and she was now on the ground catching her breath, but she also looked a little dazed. Her eyes met mine and she smiled for the first time. I told her she was safe. I told her I needed her cuffs for a citizen's arrest. She smiled and said, "I was going to shoot them, but I never got around to it." We both laughed, even though it was a very likely possibility. She winced in pain and I asked what hurts. She said, "My arm and my chest. I'm okay. I can wait. Make sure they are secure."

I grabbed her two sets of handcuffs and threw a pair to Connor. I took one pair for my bad guy. I could hear sirens and a police helicopter overhead. They had arrived as they were flying in the area. We had flipped over the bad guys, so they were face down, so we could keep an eye on them both as we went to work on the officer. They were both secure and no more trouble. The officer's backup arrived, and minutes later, there was lots more. I was just glad they could see we were the good guys, or I might have gotten a .308 round in the chest or a 9mm in the head. We were quickly surrounded, and some pointed their guns at the bad guys while others immediately set up a safety perimeter around their wounded officer. The bad guys were then flipped over, and they were searched as well as disarmed of anything that could cause harm to anyone.

Two or three police officers took over looking after each bad man and they were not our priority anymore. The injured police office was the priority now that the scene was safe and secure. The other officers immediately spread out, searched the truck for more bad guys and found drugs, a handgun, a knife, and what looked to be a bag of money. It could have been much worse if the officer had not been able to call for help. The 10-33 call would send over every officer for miles as well as tactical and other responders to assist an officer in trouble. They would drop anything they were doing and get there as fast as possible.

We then took over on the injured officer. We quickly applied field dressing to her obvious injuries. She was smiling up at us both even though she was hurt. This lady was one tough officer. She introduced herself as this was our first encounter. We had likely seen one other before but never been formally introduced. I knew, just as she knew, that she was a lucky lady. She told us it was a good thing she had some bigger brothers to fight with as a kid. They turned out to be pretty good trainers for hand-to-hand combat. I guess it's no wonder that they were all police officers now. There was no doubt in my mind she was one person you would not want to get in a fight with.

Some people radiate strength and she was one of those people. She was small and mighty and was alive today due to her training. She was fighting to live, and a few dedicated EMS staff evened up the odds. My partner called our dispatcher and updated them on our situation and additional EMS units were sent out. They would check on STARS' estimated time of arrival, as well. So far, we could handle the scene until other units arrived.

Thankfully, her injuries were neither serious nor life-threating, but she needed to have a complete assessment. She was lucky she was wearing her vest and didn't let them corner her. We quickly packaged her up on the emergency tactical stretcher and, when the first unit arrived, she was placed in the unit and we went to work. We had been notified that STARS were finishing their current call and would then meet us at the closest rural hospital. One of the other paramedics, John, took over her care in the unit. On that day John was partnered with Salt as the PCP, and now they had Connor helping them, too. They didn't need me, so I backed out, and it was then their call. My role was almost done; other than to replace the initial dressings, and write an ePCR, I just had to clean our PRU unit and it would be all over for me.

After a quick assessment, it looked like the officer had a wrist fracture, a few superficial stab wounds to her shoulder and to her hand, and one slightly troubling stab wound to her lower side. They were quickly dressed. We were quite sure it never penetrated deep enough to cause internal injuries and now was not the time to probe the injury. We arranged for a convoy and we were ready to be leave the scene in less than five minutes, headed toward the closest helipad at our local hospital.

I had quickly assessed the two bad guys who needed to be seen, but their formal care could wait until they were in custody in a controlled environment. They looked like they both had been attacked by a mountain lion. They would be sore for a few weeks and would have lots of time to heal in a jail cell. They may have outweighed her and outnumbered her, but she was tough and an experienced, combat-trained officer. They were not going to win against her easily, even if they thought they could get away with it. Today the *COPS* theme song was playing in my head: "Bad boys, bad boys, what-cha gonna do?" These guys weren't doing anything other than going to jail to sleep it off today.

On our arrival at the local hospital, STARS was just touching down. In minutes, they had her on board and were performing their preflight checks. The big chopper gained speed and they soared up and away. She had an ultrasound and extra assessment to ensure she was safe to fly before lift-off. One of her supervisors got to jump in the copter with her and would entertain her for the short flight to the nearest trauma centre. She would no doubt have a few bad moments after this day, but, all in all, she was lucky. I knew we had made a new friend for life and that felt good.

The most important thing about that day was that we had people who cared and people who were in just the right profession to help others. That day was one many of us would not forget. The outcome could have been so different, but it had worked out in our favour. Looking back, I had the right partner and we had the perfect response vehicle for the situation.

Having just the right team members makes our job easy.

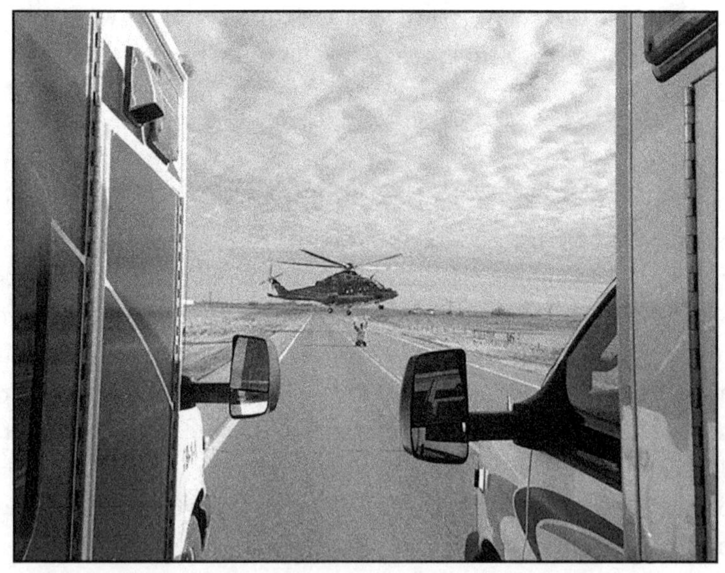

The best sight in the world. Our injured patient up and away in the hands of the STARS crew.

Chapter 7: Driving Really Does Matter

"Driver Training Requirements"

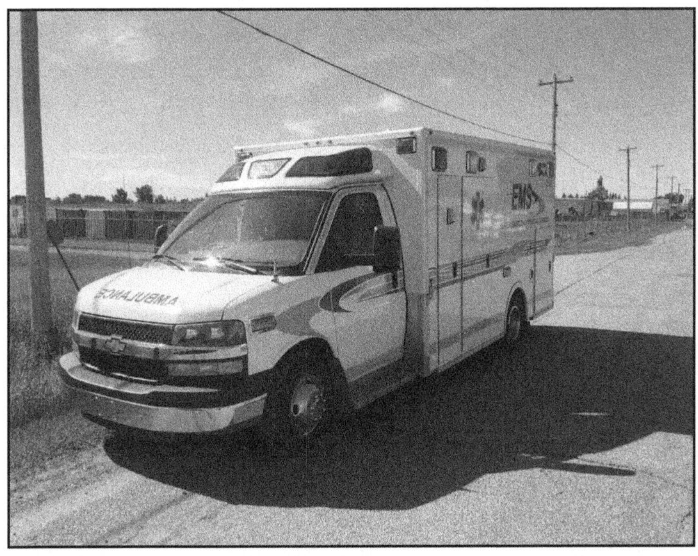

It all comes down to safety. Everything from accelerating, braking, handling and stopping a unit during an emergency— it's not the same as driving your car or truck.

The best professional EMS drivers are trained drivers. But ideal training is not always easy to get. Traditionally, the newest EMS members are EMRs and PCPs and many have no formal tactical driving experience. In an ideal EMS system, all EMS staff and students would be formally trained in driving EMS vehicles. Response units started out as simple station wagons, then evolved into vans and eventually graduated to the truck chassis with a box added for patient care. In short, the size of EMS vehicles has increased in both size and weight. The handling, braking and turning radius, as well as routine safety procedures for handling in abnormal driving situations, are much different than for a car or a normal truck. We have graduated to ambulances that are made to be ambulances right from the very start.

The driver must ensure that they are driving for the safety of themselves and their partner, first and foremost. Obviously, the patient's life is also on the line. The role of the driver is essential for the attendant who is providing care in the back. We are often busy performing treatments during the call and if you drive hard, it is difficult to perform skills in the back. I've been thrown all over in the back while trying to do my best to save a life, thinking all the while that I'll be the next one to die, all because of an inexperienced driver. It's not their fault—most times they have not been properly taught and they have no idea what it's like to function in the back unless someone shows them. Basically, whatever you do, do it slowly and try not to shake up your partner. You can't accelerate too fast, change lanes suddenly, or brake too hard, or you are likely to hurt your partner.

My favourite way to hammer this point home is by setting students up with scenarios in the back of the unit while I drive it. Once they are actively caring for their "patient," I start driving recklessly, and they will see the problem in minutes. Performing CPR while the driver is braking or turning corners too fast makes everyone in the patient compartment realize that even a little turn of the wheel can cause someone standing in the back of the open unit to lose their balance. We then teach them to verbally call bumps and corners and to give a special warning when they must brake hard. Another teaching method I use is called the "fish bowl." I take a large bowl of water and put it on the abdomen of the student who plays the role of the patient. The driver has to drive without dumping the water and making everyone wet. It is a very effective training tool!

Students learn to slow down and to drive around corners like they are professional drivers before the end of the day.

A driving course is an essential part of EMS training. Students need to see first-hand the repercussions that their driving has on everyone from the patients to the providers. They need to learn that the unit will respond differently than a smaller vehicle would when braking and taking corners. They need to experience what it's like to be a patient in the back, and then an attendant, with someone else driving recklessly. Some road situations and conditions are unavoidable and unpredictable, like pot holes and train tracks, or a driver cutting you off when you don't expect it. You need to be prepared for the fact that other drivers can be jerks, but you can do your part by driving in defensive mode to help increase the safety of everyone you are chaperoning.

It's admittedly difficult not to push the unit, especially when you're driving with your lights and siren running. The more adrenalin you release, the harder it is to drive carefully. It's an art to be able to respond to a life-and-death call safely. The art of driving is something that needs to be practiced and needs to be taught from one's very first EMS course.

Many new staff have never had the chance to drive an ambulance until after they are hired to do just that. They have never had the chance to drive an ambulance unit or anything larger than a regular-sized car or a small half-ton truck. Part of the initial driving course would be an orientation to the unit. Students would make a visual assessment of the unit and learn that the mirrors and the area needed to park are much larger. Your mirrors stick out a lot more. You're higher from the ground and this affects your centre of gravity. You are on dual tires, making your unit handle and brake differently as well.

Fortunately, many of the new units have better backup mirrors and cameras, which makes it that much easier to back up or to park.

Parking practice should ideally happen in a big parking lot with a professional driving instructor. Once new staff are comfortable in handling the unit, they can proceed to taking actual calls where they are responsible for others' lives. Often, when on a call with an inexperienced driver, I will prompt the driver from the back while I'm providing patient care, until they become accustomed to driving with a computer aided dispatch system with a live map of our response. That alone can be a distraction.

Distracted driving is a serious matter. One time we had a lady in labour about to have an imminent delivery and she was trying her best not to have the baby before we arrived at the hospital. I needed to tell the driver to hurry up, but I didn't want to worry the patient. I then resorted to texting the driver, "Please drive safe but giv'er," and he knew what I meant. I didn't want to bug him, and texting was, to me, preferable to yelling; that would just have worried the patient and her family in the back. I would have helped deliver the baby in the unit if necessary, but if we had trouble with the newborn, I would have been in over my head. This lady had some adverse history with her two previous children; both had ended up in the neonatal intensive care unit (NICU) upon delivery. I wasn't about to advise my driver to simply pull over so that I could deliver her on the side of the road unless I had no other choice.

After the vehicle orientation for the new hires we would have some fun with them. We'd take them out for a day of driving in the ambulance and get them to turn on moment's notice, or alter their speed. Back then they would have to back up with a spotter and without the use of a built-in camera in the unit. Then we would let our experienced partners take them for a drive and give them some tips in regard to driving the unit. We spent extra time with them teaching them to use the computer aided dispatch (CAD) system to help them plan their route and define their location.

They needed to learn how to get to a patient's location via the quickest route possible and had to be able to plot alternate routes using the computer-aided maps. They also needed to know about driving through construction zones when people are wearing hearing protectors and might not be able to hear them coming. Furthermore, they had to be able to handle complications such as high-traffic volume and wide loads in school zones. A good habit to get into is to always avoid school zones when in an emergency vehicle. You also wanted to stay away from congested areas if possible. Being an ambulance driver takes more skill than is immediately apparent. Driving an ambulance is an advanced art and takes a master's skill to do it well. Many of us can tell you stories of near misses that would make your heart skip a beat.

Driving simulators and watching videos of prior accidents are two of the best teaching tools, as they demonstrate why accidents occur and how best to avoid them. The number one accident sites are intersections, because you can't count on people to behave predictably. Rather, people will do what you least expect, like running a red light with the PRU in the middle of the intersection with full lights and sirens. Some people will even cut you off on purpose, so you can't get through the intersection or pass them. I was once cut off three times while on an emergency call. No matter what I did this driver would not let me pass. I was shocked. I had never had someone cut me off on purpose before while we were trying to save a life.

Fortunately, the RCMP were following me, so I simply pulled over and the RCMP took over the passing problem. I was running out of options as I could not get past or around the evil person. I was very impressed at the way the police handled the situation. They drove up and ran the person off the road and, like magic, we were free to proceed on our way to our critical patient. It was something you would never expect to have to happen, but not all people respect us. We cheered as we proceeded lights-and-siren down the highway, but it should have never needed to happen in the first place. I hope that the driver got a penalty and there were adequate demerits.

Just remember: As you approach an intersection in an emergency vehicle with your lights and siren activated, you are *asking* for the right of way. That doesn't mean that others will give it to you willingly. Also keep in mind that other emergency vehicles might be coming from other directions. For example: Many years ago, we were responding to a shooting, and as I came up to an intersection, our second responding unit was coming from a different side of town. We each knew that the other unit was being dispatched so that we could back each other up. As I entered the intersection, I needed to come to a sudden complete stop, as did the other responding unit, as we both entered the same intersection with our sirens blaring.

Luckily, we were both aware of the coincidence. They yielded to us, and we were off with them hot on our bumper. It would have been a complete tragedy to collide in an intersection with one of our corresponding units. It just goes to show you that you never own the road. "Drive to arrive alive" is a good motto for all EMS drivers regardless of the type of vehicle they are driving or why they are responding to a call. We need to leave our emotion out of the driver's seat and always consider the safety of all others as our primary reason to be in EMS.

Another time, we were dispatched to a multi-vehicle collision with up to six patients. It is common to dispatch with some uncertainly involved. It's often a vague or an uncertain initial call assessment; we are often unsure of the number of people with injuries or who needs medical care until we arrive on scene, triage, and make an overall scene assessment. I was driving, and my partner—a good friend and long-time co-worker—was mapping us to the scene and we were not wasting any time.

On route, we come to a small town and had to cross the railroad tracks. As I came up to the crossing, I could see the train in the distance and the lights had just started to flash. Then the arms started coming down. I made a calculated guess on the speed and time needed to cross and went for it. I never thought much about it until after, and then it bugged me. Often, we know lives are in jeopardy, and if we have to wait for a train, we will be stuck for five to seven minutes sometimes. It can be difficult to judge if one should take a risk or play it safe. Did I make a mistake or was it the right thing to do? The more I thought about it afterwards, the more I realized we all take risks every day. Then I thought, "What if it the train had hit us, and the other six people also died because we hadn't made it?" That would have been a total of eight lives lost. The price we could have paid was not worth it, as the price of my partner's life, plus my own, was too high of a price to pay. You're never too old to learn an important life lesson.

The lesson from that day was not needed until a year later when we were called to another very bad scene. We'd had a somewhat uneventful day with an easy call to start the day. My partner that day was Jonathan, a fine primary care paramedic (PCP) who was working hard to become an advanced care paramedic (ACP) within the coming year. That day was one I won't ever forget. Even though I had been to many train accidents, this one would forever change the way I thought, and I would truly hate train accidents for the rest of my career. We were paged to a vehicle vs train accident. On route, we could see that the long train had stopped, which was never a good sign. We initially did not know what crossing we were going to as the flag was not up and we were so quick to respond; the accident was still in the pre-call stage. In thirty seconds, the flag came up behind us, so we had to do an abrupt stop and head the other way.

We had a 50/50 chance of being right. We turned the vehicle around, and as we were turning, we could see the carnage. It was bad. It looked like a vehicle had been hit at high speed by a train, as there were pieces of the vehicle everywhere. As we pulled up, I could see activity by the side of the vehicle. There were multiple people already trying to help the injured. Bystander CPR is never a good sign when you come across an accident. It's one of the biggest predictors of a bad outcome.

Often, we have no real idea of the number of patients before we arrive on scene, and if they are dead or alive. We grabbed our monitor, ALS kits, and walked onto the scene to see what we could do. On arrival, we found a sole patient whose life was in jeopardy. There is no way that a body can take that type of impact and not be broken. If he was going to have a chance, we had to work quickly and methodically as a team, and we had to find out the reason why he was in cardiac arrest. A trauma arrest is the time to be aggressive and to get things done. High flow oxygenation, ventilation with a BVM, and aggressive IV therapy must all be applied while looking for the six deadly conditions that kill our patients in minutes. They are known also as the Lethal Six: an airway obstruction, a tension or bilateral pneumothorax, cardiac tamponade, open pneumothorax with chest wall injury, as well as a massive unilateral or bilateral hemothorax, and a flail chest are immediate, life-threatening injuries that can kill a person quickly.

This call centred on determining if any of these Lethal Six were present. With such an accident, you will usually come across some bleeding, and it will be either minor, controlled or severe. Internal bleeding can be invisible, but deadly. (In this case, it was most likely deadly external or internal bleeding judging from the mechanism of injury.) What amazed me was how much blood someone could lose and still fight to stay alive.

Our biggest priority on arrival, is to treat the deadly complications that can be treated. All we can hope to do is find the biggest threats to the life and try to reduce the stress to the body if possible. As you soon learn, sometimes you can "stay and play," which means stay on scene and try to intervene with our advanced life support (ALS) skills and sometimes you need to run. On this day, we needed to run—or load our patient into the unit—and drive as fast as possible to the local emergency room so the experts could help us try and save a life.

On this call we tried everything from BLS to ALS treatments. A local volunteer firefighter/paramedic arrived to help us, plus we got another volunteer firefighter to drive for us. Everything that could possibly be done was being done. We knew we were fighting a losing battle, but for part of the transport and for a short time in hospital we maintained a pulse. We performed some heroic measures, but in the end, we could not change the outcome. It was a hard day for many people: the train conductor, rail staff, police, volunteer firefighters and all others on scene. The hospital staff had an especially hard job; in addition to dealing with the patient after we arrived, they had to inform the family that their loved one didn't make it. Nobody involved that day was left untouched by the tragedy.

There was no overcoming the number of horrific internal injuries. What amazes me is how much blood someone can lose and still fight to stay alive. Conversely, the next patient we see can have very little blood loss and be asystole almost right away. After the call, we all pitched in to help clean up the mess. It really made me appreciate just how suddenly tragedy can take a life. I thought back to the other call where I made the decision to try to beat the train, and it hit me that the risk is never worth the potential outcome. You just can't keep pushing fate without something tragic eventually occurring. After a few hours, I called my partner from the previous call and apologized for crossing in front of the train. It was just not worth the risk.

When you think you have the art of driving an ambulance mastered, try responding in the PRU on your own. It becomes progressively more difficult as you respond to more serious calls. When you become the PRU operator, you must master the art of multitasking, including talking on the radio, running the computer, knowing the limits of the vehicle, and being aware of the road conditions and your own limits, as well. Not only are you responsible for your patient's, co-workers' and your own safety, but you are also responsible for the safety of everyone else on the road. Having to make complex decisions while driving an emergency vehicle, operating a computer-aided dispatch display and communicating to Dispatch is not something that can be mastered overnight. But with time, you will be able to do it without much thought.

Weather and road conditions are so variable. The one thing you can't change is road conditions and they are greatly affected by the current weather. Snow, sleet, freezing rain and high winds all put our driving skills to the test. Many people assume that because you're driving an ambulance, you're trained, but until recently, driver training was the exception and *not* the standard. Driving in high-top module ambulances is not the same as driving a car or a truck for many reasons. The wind can be so strong that it threatens to tip your vehicle. Everyone needs to know the roads they are driving and anticipate challenges before they occur. Even the best drivers can have a bad day driving.

The toughest conditions to drive in are snow and freezing rain. Temperatures around freezing can make the roads very dangerous and driving much more difficult. The trick to driving on bad roads is to practice your driving techniques with a driving instructor first. It goes without saying that when the roads are poor, lower speeds will keep you safer. Never assume roads are perfect, as that is a mere fairytale. The dual tires on bigger units are helpful for dispersing weight but make traction and handling in snow and water challenging. The most important thing to know is that heavier units require much more room to stop then you would think.

There are huge differences between driving in urban and rural locations. The one aspect of driving that we all learn to master is how to navigate around other vehicles in a safe manner. Regardless of whether you are driving in small towns or busy cities with lights and sirens, people might not be accommodating or willing to give you the right of way. That's the real driver's test. Some people just don't care about the need to get a patient to the hospital because it interferes with whatever their plans are. That's the world we now live in, so "drive to arrive alive" is the most anyone can ask from you (especially your partner and your patient).

This chapter has only scratched the surface of the topic of professional driving. The requirements to drive effectively are so much more detailed and extensive than what can be discussed here. We are all part of the team and, just like every team, some people will be better at driving than others. Like any skill, some people are able to master it and long before others. Just remember, you can save many lives over the years but it's important to understand that you can just as easily take a life in seconds with one mistake. You won't get a second chance, so take driving very seriously and always drive defensively.

A sign in a local fire hall where I did a lot of training comes to mind. It was signed by Alan Brunacini, Incident Commander, and it simply read:

- ***We will risk our lives a lot, in a highly calculated and controlled manner, to protect a salvageable life.***
- ***We will risk our lives a little, in a highly calculated and controlled manner, to protect salvageable property.***
- ***We will not risk our lives at all to protect lives or property that are already lost.***

These three statements apply to many things we do in the EMS profession. There can be no mistaking the reason and logic in these words, not only as they apply to the EMS professional but also to all activities of daily living. Despite how carefully we respond to situations and no matter what risks we take, the need to be vigilant in matters of safety remains constant. It is important to take a moment and consider the risk in any situation—that there is a time for us not to take chances or risk our own lives or especially those of our partners. I have learned through experience that we are never done learning if we simply take the time to reflect on our calls, no matter how many calls or years we have worked. We can all learn something new if we take the time to notice the things around us.

The best takeaway, my friends, is to be diligent about your safety and stay safe. Always look for hazards, always be a mentor, and always do your best on every call. Finally, never ever forget we are forever students in emergency medical services, for our career can be and often is a lifelong career. Accept the personal along with the professional challenges and help us in our goal to make our profession even stronger.

Chapter 8: Protocol vs. Medical Guidelines

"Patient Care vs. the System Rules"

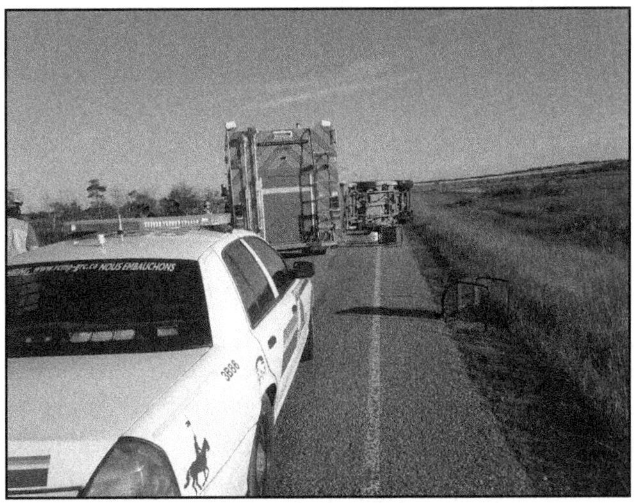

Police and Fire – keeping us all safe

It's impossible to accurately predict the initial patient presentations after a 911 call is made and we are dispatched. We never know the particulars of the hazards on scene or potential threats we may walk into on certain calls. Many times, the dispatchers can get a sense of the scene and can forewarn us that the scene is not as safe as it could be, and we will stage accordingly until the police can ensure our safety. In the interval between the time of the call and our arrival, a patient's condition can go from unstable to stable and then back again. Often, the outcome can be positively affected with the right interventions from bystanders or first responders. Other times, as

I learned many years ago, the perpetrators can come back after our arrival. There is no guarantee of safety in the EMS world.

Often, lives can be saved by the first responders who arrive on scene and intervene before the closest EMS unit can arrive. EMS is often slowed by parameters like distance and limited speed on roads, not to mention road conditions and the ability to access the patient easily. EMS is also faced with system limitations; that is, we must follow certain rules and other legalities while we perform our job. For example, there are rules limiting student performance: local and provincial protocol and American Heart and Stroke (AHA) regulations, and they are never the same when it comes to patient care. The real test comes when we find ourselves sitting in the hospital hallway or stuck in a little room, so the public is not aware of our delayed transfer of care in urban centres. Thankfully in rural centres, that is not a problem.

The rules are ridiculously complex for students. We have the school's way, the local way, the preceptor's way, the provincial way and what is published in the textbooks. The textbooks have guidelines that may contradict the school's protocol, the preceptors may have individual preferences and there can be local habits and traditions, which may or may not be in keeping with provincial regulations. All these factors have merit depending upon the circumstance. When new staff start, they need support and we need to ensure they are mentored properly to make up for their lack of experience. That is why we should start talking about treatment options on the way to calls. It is common for partners to talk about the call on the way and make a game plan. I would usually arrive on a call with about three plans of attack, depending on the initial assessment. If the dispatch information matched the call information, we already knew if it was going to be a "load and go" or "stay and play" situation. If there were any mortal threats, we altered our treatments. Then we performed the rest of the care, or as much of it as possible, while we were on route to the closest emergency room (ER).

Many times, we are trying to please multiple players as we try to save a life, all while following separate rules or guidelines for each set of practitioners. First responders, who are trying to do their job, function under one set of guidelines, then along comes the prehospital care providers who have been trained at different levels by different schools. They must then work within the guidelines of the local service, all while working toward the goal of getting the patient to the hospital in an improved state. Finally, the hospital administering the receiving care can either be amazing or less than stellar. There are always so many unknown circumstances that one must constantly be ready to intervene or alter one's plans to best suit the patient's overall care.

Often, crews need to adapt their care parameters to compensate for a patient's condition, and then they have to decide on the best transport options, all while watching out for common transportation complications. The LP-15 monitor with its constant CO2, SpO2, BP and heart-rate monitoring, allows crews to intervene before a patient goes into severe distress or deteriorates. We often need to decide on the best care options before arrival at the receiving hospital and seriously weigh the pros and cons of the treatments. We first need to "do no harm." That has to be the golden rule in every situation, regardless of circumstances.

Occasionally, two paramedics have such great chemistry when they partner up that they form a "dream duo." Today I was thinking about my past calls with my old partner Sarah who was in her last semester of paramedic school. God, how I miss her kind and gentle soul. Then there was the legendary "Salt and Pepper," a pair of inseparable primary care paramedics (PCPs). People rarely used their real names, but they were some of my greatest past students and they were one of the best duos I've ever seen. They just fit together like no other two people on earth. Their strengths were many and their weakness were few as a team. I was humbled to know God made such special people to work in EMS and I would do everything in my power to keep them safe. From time to time, I would have the privilege of working with them.

We started our tour together with our regular unit check. It was amazing how many drugs or medical devices we could stock in one unit. I loved taking the newest staff through the units, but on this occasion, Salt was doing the unit check and Pepper was checking drugs with me. As we went through the medications, we engaged in a very good verbal debate: When to "stay and play" and use our ALS skills and when to "load and go" and make a run for the closest ER. The answer is neither simple, nor easy. The best paramedics in the world all have trouble with this common dilemma. If you have a partner with whom you're on the same page as far as treatment options, it's easier to decide most of the time. For example, if a patient needs an operating room (OR) or immediate critical care intervention, it's a good time to head for a hospital.

On our first day shift, we were called to a small-town hospital to help in the local ER. On arrival, we found a thirty-five-year-old male in acute respiratory distress, hypotensive and uncooperative. I took one look at Salt and Pepper and said, "Let's go to work, ladies." The day just got a lot more complicated for everyone. This would be the best type of transfer to learn from and for all of us to share experiences from. By mentoring the PCPs today on this very difficult call, the next difficult call they had, they would be one step ahead of the rest of the class. There are many lessons you can't teach in class, but during a critical care transfer you can quickly share your wisdom and make sure the lessons of the day are not in vain.

As usual I went through all the possible treatment options as we received the dispatch information. I had the plan made up long before we arrived on scene. We needed to know if we had backup coming or if STARS could fly in, and where the best hospital to transport to was as the call progressed. If you practiced and planned for any situation and it never happened, you were lucky, but you always needed to plan for the worst and pray for the best. It was a good habit to get the new members on the team thinking out loud. I loved knowing that we were both thinking about the most common complications we might encounter and how to avert or prevent a medical disaster in the making.

One thing about emergency medicine is it's hard to teach or get people to understand that protocol doesn't apply perfectly to every patient. The hardest part to teach staff is to treat your patient and not just go by protocol, as you can have a patient who meets the guidelines, but in the beginning the cause or underlining conditions are truly unknown. Doing the right thing means treating each patient as an individual case.

This was the verbal report we received that day: A gentleman had apparently just shown up with some friends who had dropped him off and disappeared. The history of events was unknown. It could possibly have been a chemical exposure, drug ingestion, or shock from any number of conditions. Often, when a patient is in trouble, the sympathetic nervous system is running on maximum and any confusion or lack of cooperation is then from lack of basic oxygenation, lack of brain perfusion and a buildup of unwanted chemical waste in the blood or respiratory system.

We started with the ABC approach and stabilized the patient as best as we could. Cleared the airway first, then assisted with breathing, and then worked on circulation. After applying the LP-15 monitor along with its sensors, we had his temperature, assessed his blood sugar, and performed a constant 4-lead and a baseline12-lead to help decide the most likely differential diagnosis. Then we could better isolate the real reason the patient was in trouble. If we just treated one condition and used one protocol on a sick person, we would have trouble keeping them out of harm's way for very long.

We planned the care right from the start. I said, "He's sick; let's go to war." Salt was all over the monitor, Pepper was looking after the oxygen therapy and IV access and I was busy getting the story straight while assessing the patient from head to toe. We called out our findings as soon as we noted them. The outlook was looking worse as the seconds added up. The summary was essentially hypoxia, hypotension, and an altered level of consciousness (LOC), which was not surprising. We all knew we were in trouble.

The patient was essentially trying his best to die, and we needed to come up with a game plan to avert the pending disaster. I had no clue what started that particular train wreck, but I had an idea how to stop it. We had a little huddle. Today I was the quarterback and tomorrow one of them would be one step closer to taking over. The quick plan was to establish an advanced airway, administer additional fluid boluses, then add IV vasopressors to improve circulation. Then we would have the patient packaged and out the door. We had secured a receiving ICU bed, but we needed a live patient to be awarded that special bed.

We consulted the critical care physician, and it was decided that we would stay and stabilize, and they would try to send STARS to the scene, but within two minutes, we were told they were not able to come as they were on a flight. Plan B was going to be our unit, our staff and something we referred to as "diesel therapy." We contacted our dispatcher and we got the BLS transfer unit to come help us stabilize the patient and get him to the hospital sooner than later. It would be Connor and Julie to the rescue. We needed something to change our patient's presentation for the better. So far it was looking bad. We had a few tricks up our sleeves, though; namely, some very powerful medications. We would try to buy us a little time. Any extra time we could get was a good thing today.

In no time we had extra IVs established and running wide open and had secured an advanced airway despite the precarious state of this sick patient. A medicinal miracle and he was asleep. I wondered if it was going to be the last time he would ever talk to anyone, and we still had no idea why he was in such extreme distress. Our initial intravenous vasopressor agents had not been that effective.

We added sodium bicarbonate for a severe metabolic acidosis, with no improvement. The chest X-ray was technically terrible but looked like a very bad case of pneumonia. The blood work came back and indicated a severe infection, and the IV antibiotics were already running. We got him out alive, but all in all, it was not an ideal transfer. We needed holy water, but I was fresh out of any other suggestions.

We initiated the transfer. Connor was the pilot of our unit, with the rest of us in the back scrambling to keep the patient alive. But no matter what we did, his BP would not improve, and it was so low it was not even close to normal. When your BP is 68/38 and your heart rate is 48 BPM and you need extra medication to stimulate the heart, it basically means you're in huge trouble. We even added an epinephrine infusion and it made no real improvement. We were wasting no time on the transfer tonight.

I began to believe that we were not going to be able to save him. We were flying toward the best help in the world with our wheels just touching the ground, but it was not looking like we were going to make it. His oxygen level was still terribly low, and his BP had worsened to 62/32. The CO2 level was also low at eighteen, which meant terrible perfusion. We were ventilating twelve times a minute with positive end expiratory pressure, but his oxygenation was only 80-84%. His core temperature was also low at 34.6 °C. The differential diagnosis ranged from bilateral pneumonia to septic shock to drug overdose, or ARDS—possibly a combination of them all. If I was a betting man I would have said it was a case of adult respiratory distress syndrome (ARDS), which is as serious as it gets in many people trying to die. Combine that with a septic patient and the end results are very bad. Death was pulling him backwards and we were trying to drive ahead. The angel of death was winning this battle despite our best intentions.

We performed constant and repeated evaluations, and we constantly changed or added extra treatments. For every bad vital sign, we added something chemically to push the extremes out of a sick heart. About ten minutes before we arrived at the receiving hospital, the patient went into ventricular tachycardia (VT) with no palpable pulse. Salt and Pepper were all over it. One of them charged the LP-15 to 200 joules, and the other grabbed an epinephrine preload. Julie did CPR, just as well as the mechanical machines, and Connor kept the ride as smooth as possible despite the traffic around us.

I knew he would be pushing the unit to its limits, but he was one of those drivers who made you feel safe. Our guardian angels were on our side that day, regardless of the outcome. We were going to lose the battle, at least in my mind, but I was afraid to say that out loud. Somedays you just need to try and keep your mind positive and fight away the negative thoughts.

As the team leader in the back, I was constantly looking for reasons to change therapy options to improve the patient's condition. We had been doing our best to avert any changes that could lead to a cardiac arrest, for once it occurred, the chance of saving his life would be dismal at best. We always need to know we are making the right changes in patient care without causing more harm, which is not easy. All we could do was to perform good CPR and give the heart a few minutes to reset itself, if possible.

After about two minutes of the epinephrine circulating, we shocked him one more time and the pulse returned. The ideal medication for a cardiac arrest might not have been adrenalin, but it was what we used. Sometimes nothing is more effective in adult patients than good old CPR. If the body needed adrenalin to keep going, it meant the inner reserves were depleted.

I thought about anything we might be missing, and we added a few extra ampules of sodium bicarbonate just to help the acidotic state, thinking it could not hurt us now. An acidotic state was not something we would normally correct without the right laboratory test in the ambulance, which was not available at the time. We only had the initial laboratory test from the original hospital to guide us, and it was not much help. STARS or the flight crews had a blood chemical analyzer, but it wasn't present in most ground units. A chemical analyzer would have made our job so much more accurate than just guessing, but it wasn't something we could change.

As the seconds ticked past, our patient was still holding on . . . but just. I was coming up with some good one-liners to keep everyone from getting more stressed, but they were mostly falling flat on this day. We all knew we were fighting a losing battle. God knows how proud I was looking at the faces of our new EMS warriors. No matter the odds, they kept the faith and never quit or even suggested we were losing, even though we all knew it in our hearts. They just kept working like a machine.

The reality is that the human body is very complex, and health is not something we should ever take for granted. The more I learn, the more I realize we are not as smart as we think we are. It is fascinating how negative and positive feedback loops work in the human body, and the fact that our body has such delicate receptor sites, unique receptors and organs that can compensate despite the harmful things that we do to our body. It makes me wonder if someday we might have ultrasound scanners and essential laboratory tests available in all units. Maybe then we will have better luck when trying to keep the angel of death out of the unit.

When we arrived at the intensive care unit (ICU), I was sweating as I silently prayed for one more miracle from modern medicine. Our patient was on borrowed time already, and we had no more to offer from our treatment options. No matter who our patient was or why he was so sick, we wanted a good outcome for him, regardless of the circumstances. It was humbling to know everyone worked so hard on him with no expectations other than to complete their shift and to do their very best. I will never get over the fact that in health care we work so hard for our patients, who are often people we don't know, have never seen before and will most likely never see again. We bend the rules, we take chances all to save a lives day in and day out. That's who we are and that is something that is so special about first responders, be they police, firefighters, EMS or other health care staff.

Everyone on the team assumes some of the responsibility for making sure the patient has the best chance of survival. The staff quickly step into their roles and they assume them with passion and with dedication. The fact that there are people who are dedicated to helping others at high risk, despite having to make many personal sacrifices, makes me so proud. The true dedication is seen in the ICU staff as they approach a critically ill patient and how they rapidly assume responsibility of the patient's care. The ICU staff have wisdom beyond belief. This day was not unlike others. The ICU staff quickly assumed our patient's care after assessing our interventions and went to work augmenting our ALS care: inserting central lines, doing a portable chest X-ray and an array of essential diagnostic laboratory tests. We grabbed our equipment and made it out of the ICU intact. As we walked out of there, we all looked at the patient to wish him well. We had done all we could do, and the rest was up to the critical care specialist. We silently cheered as a team as we walked toward the elevator. We had done it.

The patient's next battle was not ours. Next up was time for some coffee and a debriefing on the way home. While standing in line at Tim's for my coffee, a younger man humbly walked up to our crew and said, "Thank you for all you do," smiled and shook our hands, then turned and walked away. That one act of kindness made me realize that hope comes when you least expect it. There is still hope left for humanity; with hope we have a chance and with a single chance we can make a difference.

We would have some high moments and some sullen moments as we thought about the call. Our unit was a mess and we decided to stay out of service until we could restock and do a deep clean because there had been so many unknowns on this call. We didn't want to risk spreading any germs. I gladly sat in the back and sipped on my coffee as I did the ePCR finalization right away, while my trusted crew got us all safely home.

I would say that the takeaway lesson from this day was: If you're not sure what to do, never be afraid to call for help early. We try to decide in seconds if a patient is "sick or not sick," and with that decision made, it is easier to package and initiate transport early. Sometimes, it's better to transport and decide the best care on route or on arrival to the receiving centre. You can never go wrong by performing BLS skills; BLS, along with diesel therapy to get you to your closest hospital, is as great an option as any on most days.

For new staff in our profession, it's good to be up to date on protocols, but it's more important to know that proper patient care assessment and interviewing skills are priceless. Finally, the last thing to remember is that we are but a team. No matter our individual roles, the other co-responders also have their unique roles and at the end of the day we need each other. As we pulled into our base that day, I was never so happy to see the other crew waiting to help us clean and restock our unit. Being able to share the day with other dedicated staff members allowed me to sleep well that night. No matter the outcome, we all did our best that day and that is all anyone can ever ask for.

Our lifesavers are only ever just a phone call away.

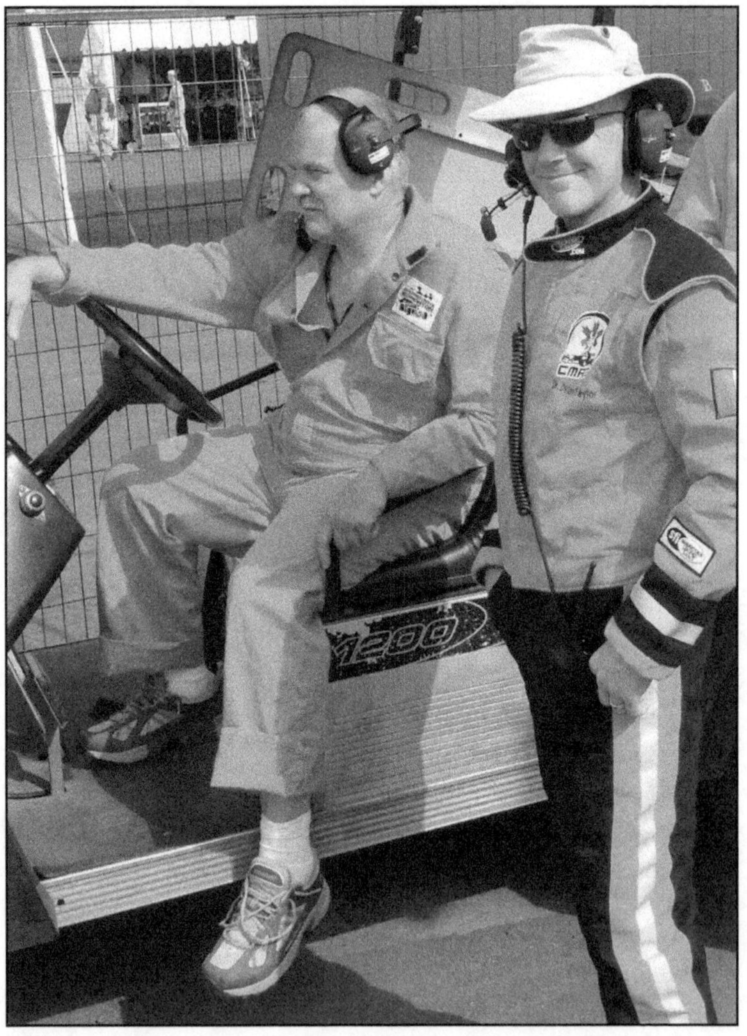

We can learn the most from people we truly trust and respect

Chapter 9: Making the Right Decision

"Common Sense vs. Wisdom"

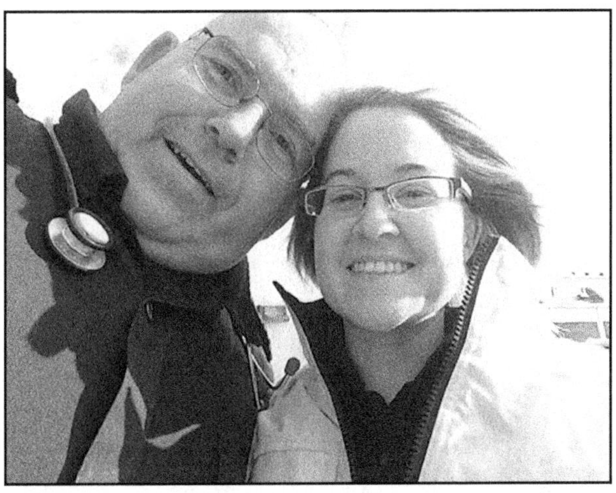

The one thing in life you can't always predict are the consequences of your decisions for the future. I have been on many calls in my lifetime, and the voice of reason and logic is one that you can't ignore. In EMS, we often want to perform heroic skills, but at the end of the day it does no good if we don't perform basic life support (BLS) skills first. Furthermore, it does no good if we mistreat a patient due to a lack of understanding of the underlying injury or illness.

We need to use our wisdom and our intuition to head down the right treatment pathway. Often the presentation of a situation or an event is not as clear as we would like it to be. In these times we must use common sense along with our assessment skills, monitors, and SAMPLE history to make the best decisions in providing the best emergency care possible. There are times when there is no visible answer to the problem. We occasionally walk into a medical disaster and are missing so much information that it's hard to make even an educated guess as to what started the chain of events. That's when common sense takes over. On a bad day, all we can hope for is to make the patient better than they were before our arrival.

The art of making good decisions comes from experience, and you can't get that from any textbook. Experience and wisdom come from doing repeated emergency calls and making a few bad decisions along the way. Teaching a student to make the right decision on any one type of call is not easy. I have repeatedly been reminded that students should only learn enough to be successful at their current level. I would often teach my students extra material, but the problem with that is that students are always being challenged by other practitioners. New employees are judged for their lack of knowledge, even if it's above the level of expertise of those judging them. Although it is important that BLS providers and primary care paramedics (PCP) adhere to protocol, they also need to understand that they provide just one level of care on a continuum.

On any given day, they can work with a partner who has more education and more experience, and they will need to be competent. They will often need to give a report to a nurse, paramedic, or physician, and therefore they need extra knowledge to understand the basic care required. They will often arrive to a call and find a patient in a very unstable condition from many possible complications. You will never get two calls that will have the same presentation. You will never regret learning too much, but you will regret not being able to do enough to save a life.

A new employee needs to know their scope of practice as thoroughly as possible, but also must know what else could be done for additional patient care, even if it isn't protocol or is beyond your level of care. Often there are treatment and assessment skills not included under protocol. Comprehensive patient care is not just black and white. There are grey areas where we must alter our care, attempt the best treatments despite limited resources, and lack of medications or equipment on our ambulances. Some days, we simply assess the patients we are called to help, and then we must analyze our findings, while monitoring vital signs. We then need to come up with an idea of which underlying conditions are most likely to be present. At that point, we can decide the most appropriate course of action and do our best with what we can see or understand. Then we constantly reassess, intervene and adjust our therapies as required. The best outcomes come from the days we are working as a team. Along with that, we need to be flexible and simply remain honest with others and ourselves. You are only one part of the team, regardless of your level of training or your years of service. It is never wrong to admit that you're not sure or don't know what is wrong with the patient and simply package them up and take them to a higher level of care where they can be properly treated.

In time, most students and new staff understand that guidelines are somewhat flexible for good reason. It's all part of lifelong learning. The best part of being in EMS for a long time is you get to see and work with your success stories. Over the years, I have had many success stories as new partners.

One day, I woke up and was so happy knowing it would be another day spent helping others. The day started out with a bang. I had just walked in the front door of the base and there was a call waiting. The night crew was just coming in the door from their last call and I said to them, "Don't worry, it's ours." I quickly signed out some medications and put them in my pouch. This is what is commonly referred to as a "narcotic pouch," although they typically contain much more than just narcotics. I call it our secret weapon against suffering, pain, anger and hostility. I often said we had more medications than people had anger, and I meant it. Laughing and a good sense of humour were also great weapons against pain and suffering when used appropriately.

A good paramedic knows when and when not to use controlled medications and how much to administer at any given time. One must weigh the pros and cons of using almost every medication. I grabbed my radio, ensured it was turned on, and then all I needed was a partner. Then I saw my partner's smiling face come in from the bay; it was Pepper. She was like a shining light from heaven. I just hopped my bad luck never corrupted her pure spirit. I knew we would have fun today no matter what the world threw in our direction. She had already signed us into the computer-aided dispatch system in the unit and we were ready to fly.

Pepper had our unit all ready to go. She had come in early and had done the unit checks and was more than ready for work. I said, "You navigate the CAD and I'll drive," to which she said, "Deal." She passed me my favourite Timmy's blend and we were off, lights and sirens blaring, as soon as we left the parking lot. Our day started off as well as it could. Now only time would determine how the rest of our day went.

"Dear God," I prayed, "please watch over us as we hit the highway." All we knew was that we were responding to a two-vehicle MVC, the rest was unknown. Backup had been dispatched and would be a few minutes behind us. We shook hands as we passed the posted speed limit, with sirens and lights our primary protectors. Today we had the positive edge over others as we knew we could, and would, work as a team no matter what we faced. I had a feeling that this call was not going to be a typical call, so I pushed the limits to get there a little faster. Our co-responders were all on their way, but I knew we would most likely be the first to arrive at the scene. It would give us a few minutes to perform a quick triage and then update the other responders.

It was a about a twenty-minute trip, which meant that we had time to prepare our thoughts, arrange backup units and add additional co-responders. I thought carefully to ensure we had covered all the important parts before we arrived. I then said, "I have some good news and I have some bad news." Pepper looked at me with a puzzled look as I said, "You are in charge." She just smiled at me and said, "You're kidding," as she punched me lightly in the shoulder. I said, "Okay, this one is mine but the next one is yours." I was just trying to lessen her anxiety as it was my several hundredth MVC and only her second. I would keep her safe and she would watch my back. We would get through this one no matter the trials we would face.

Just before we arrived on scene, we were updated. We now had three patients and one suspected deceased. If there was only one victim and one deceased on arrival (DOA), we might have been able to attempt interventions, but the odds were against us today. Some days we are meant to lose a life.

So, before we even started out, we were minus one already. It was time to put on our serious battle mask. We would not back down no matter what we faced. We had local volunteer firefighters, two additional EMS units, and the PRU on the way. We were notified that STARS had been called and would be airborne shorty. We would send the most critical patients, one or two, to an urban trauma team. We would need to determine care for the other one on the scene, as well as decide what we would do in the unit or on route to hospital. Transportation decisions would be made on scene as a collective of crews, determined by the injuries and needs of each patient on our arrival. The best transport crew would quickly be decided, as well as the best place to send them. The rest was easy. All we had to do was save a life using the ATLS mentality. Advanced trauma life support skills and lessons refined over the years would help us provide the best patient care possible. We would get Pepper some very good trauma experience today. I just prayed my tradition of bad luck stopped before this day was over. We needed a good outcome and we would make it happen in spite of the odds against us.

The triage process would be straightforward. It would simply be a question of "who can we save" and "who should we put our efforts into as a worthwhile cause." We could not afford to expend effort on someone who had stopped breathing and had no pulse today. I quickly said to my partner, "We got this one, girl." We shook hands and gave each other a high five. It was game on. It was time to save a life or two. We just needed to look after the mess until our backup arrived. Today we were first on scene. As we pulled up, we could see one vehicle mangled on the highway and one in the ditch. One person was lying across the centre line. That would most likely be the deceased person. Being ejected from a moving, rolling vehicle almost never ends well. Seat belts, airbags and staying inside the patient compartment is a good idea in almost every accident.

We parked crosswise to protect the person or the body with our unit and close enough to deflect traffic if needed, so no one could run over them or us. We jumped out and separated. I would take one of the vehicles and Pepper would check the other one. I grabbed the ALS airway bag and Pepper had the trauma kit. We would each quickly assess and evaluate the patients in each vehicle. Then we would collectively decide the best treatment and transport options. The person on the road was also my patient but with one look at him from a few feet away, I knew he was already deceased. So, I kept walking to the vehicle I was to assess, knowing some family was about to have a bad day.

I arrived at my vehicle and found one person unconscious and struggling for every breath in the passenger seat. From the look of the cab, one person had been ripped out of the driver's seat, most likely the deceased person. The face in the front passenger seat was unrecognizable, and the chest was also a broken mess. I would call it a bilateral flail chest. This patient had two of the most common deadly injuries. I looked hard to see if I knew her; it was impossible to know for sure, but something about her looked familiar.

We had no good access to the surviving patient in the mangled wreckage. The roof needed to be removed. I could only get my hands in a little bit while trying to assess the patient. Today, we had everything working against us all. I decided to insert an artificial airway and then decompress her chest with big needles. My access was so limited that it was almost impossible to do anything. I would try my best anyway. The options were limited.

I attempted to use a bag valve mask (BVM) to ventilate her broken chest and lungs, but it was too small of a space. I had slipped in an artificial airway as I first assessed her, but it wasn't great. The patient needed suctioning, which was almost impossible in the small space. If only we had a few more inches of room we could perform our skills, but when the vehicle rolled, the roof had crushed her, and that was probably the reason for the severe facial injuries and significant chest injuries. I slipped high-flow nasal prongs onto her face. It wasn't ideal, but it was oxygen; for the moment it would have to suffice. I then turned and got my partner's attention. I asked her what she had, already knowing we were both in trouble.

Pepper had two patients in her vehicle. One had suspected chest and abdomen injuries but was awake and in moderate distress in the passenger seat. The driver was unconscious with a suspected head injury, as well as a broken femur and arm. We determined that two of the patients needed STARS, and the advanced care that their trauma teams offered. Based on the mechanism of injury (MOI), all three patients warranted trauma teams, but that was not going to be possible with the resources at hand. The best we could do was to arrange on-scene care and to rush the most injured to the hospital via the fastest transport method. All three people in our hands needed much more care then we could provide. We were capable of many basic and advanced life support skills, but we were neither surgeons nor critical care intensivists, and we had no blood products available. Even with the best critical care physicians and the best surgeons in the world, the outcomes might be less than ideal. Some days we needed a miracle.

We determined that STARS could take one patient from the scene and then come back for the second one once we diverted to the closest hospital to stabilize with some expert help. The third patient could simply bypass via an ALS unit with a few extra staff helping during transport. We notified dispatch of our options and then got to work on a solution. The backup units and STARS staff would be notified of the awaiting chaos. The biggest immediate issue was that we still had to cut the people out of the vehicles, which takes time. Today our patients' golden hour was rapidly being depleted.

We had to wait for the firefighters to cut the surviving patients out and that was just the way it was. Some days, we could sneak the broken patients out a hole in the carnage but today that wasn't possible. Pepper had assessed her patients and I had assessed mine. It was a debate who might make it and only time would declare the winners and losers of this disaster. Pepper and I both did the best we could while we waited for backup to come, as we tried covering the basics; stopping any visible bleeding, airway care, breathing adjuncts and IV access was a start for the surviving patients today. We had each other on our minds as we went to work. Pepper would not let me down and I was not going to leave her stranded. We shared our ALS equipment and did what we were trained to do and that was all anyone could ask from us. Nothing was going to stop us from trying to save a life but the patient's own will to live. If only they could hang on for a little more time we would change the destiny of destruction.

In the distance, we could hear backup coming. I radioed them and set up a plan. The PRU supervisor, Greg, was going to set up in the first arriving unit for Pepper's patient, and the one patient I had could go in our unit and we would try our best to stabilize him. The third unit would take over the care of the more stable patient. STARS could toss a coin and take either of the critical patients. It was time to extricate and take our chances with room to effectively work. We would then see who would make it and who would not. After we moved some of the most critical patients, they could simply start bleeding and decompensate into cardiac arrest in mere minutes. But we had no choice but make our first move. If it went badly, we would know in seconds and we could also react as our patient's condition changed.

In minutes, fire was setting up and I would soon have a patient to work on. As we waited, the patient appeared to suddenly stop breathing. I knew she was going into cardiorespiratory arrest, and I still had no room to effectively work. If only I had some room. I grabbed the surgical airway kit. I had no other options, I inserted a surgical airway as the fire crews were setting up. I then inserted bilateral decompression needles in her flail segments and tried to ventilate her. It was a little better than expected, but not much. The fire crews worked around me. In minutes, they had enough of an opening so that we could slide her out. This was what we needed, but by this time I was sure it was too late.

She went straight onto a spine board and into the unit. There was no pulse detected, so chest compressions were immediately started. Blood was coming out of both needles in her chest. The BVM fit onto our surgical cricothyroidotomy; I normally would have tried to intubate, but today it wasn't possible. Maybe we should have inserted the chest decompression needles first, but I truly could not see or get a good enough look to decide the best care. In hindsight, it might have been a better idea. I just don't know or think it would have mattered. The simple fact of the day was that the injuries were lethal to start with, despite our interventions. You can't defeat the laws of physics even with a seat belt and an airbag in certain crashes.

The ventilations went in but not easily. The patient's chest had been crushed and, as I suspected, she had massive internal injuries. We had two IVs in right away and they were running wide open. One ampule of adrenalin (1:10000) was inserted as per protocol. By the time we got the monitor on her, she was in asystole. Everything that could go wrong was going wrong. Meanwhile, the STARS crew were landing beside us. They could help me with trying to rule out the deadly dozen and then our efforts would be terminated. I could see the extra crews helping Pepper, as well. I just hoped she was having better luck than I was so far. I felt bad as we never really got to work together. We had good intentions. But in a disaster, good intentions could destroy the potential best outcomes. In no time, I had a STARS physician at my side helping me. The other STARS crew went to help Pepper. We went through the motions of trying to save the patient, but it was futile. The patient was pronounced dead in short order, so we went and helped with the other two survivors. Now we were minus two lives and we had not even left the scene yet.

The second survivor was also in critical condition, and multiple rescuers were required to get her packaged and stabilized for a flight to the awaiting trauma team. The third patient was also stabilized and taken by ground to the closest hospital. STARS was to return as quickly as they could and transport that patient as well. I could see Pepper was working well with the other crews and any intimidation she'd felt about providing trauma care was gone. This call was a very complex call but a great learning opportunity for a new staff member.

With the extra help of all the staff on the scene, the second person was stabilized and packaged in a very rapid format and methodical order. In a very short time, the patient was loaded onto the helicopter stretcher, and they were getting ready for takeoff. Pepper and I had reunited and gave each other a huge hug. We had done it. The extra staff and the firefighters gathered, and we watched the chopper take off, turn into the wind and then rapidly climbed away. That part never got boring. It was one more successful call for us despite the losses. I was sort of disappointed with the care we'd been able to provide, but I also knew it was not our fault. Some days we are not meant to have a great outcome. We can change destiny but only when it is meant to be challenged. As the chopper climbed away, they eventually disappeared into the clouds.

We picked up our equipment and got everything loaded into our unit. The RCMP were on scene, performing the initial investigation. The local coroner had also arrived, and we needed permission to leave and drop the deceased off at the local ER, who would then arrange to transport our deceased patient to the provincial coroner's office. It was rare for us to pronounce someone in our unit, as then it became part of the crime scene and we could not leave without authorization. It seemed strange to sit and talk about the call beside the body in the unit. So, we sat on the shoulder of the road and watched the world go by instead. We shared the stories of our own adventures trying to save lives today. I told Pepper about my attempt at patient access with no luck. There simply was no room to do much. She shared with me her quick surveys and what she found.

No matter how much we wanted to do, with limited access, we'd both simply had to wait it out. It's so frustrating when you need to go to work but can't. In retrospect, maybe we should have changed patients. Being that Pepper was of a smaller build, she might have had more success accessing my patient. Sometimes you get so focused on what is in front of you and forget to look at the bigger picture. It's nobody's fault but it happens just the same.

I was fixated on the thought of why this accident had to happen in the first place. We need to prevent the disasters we can at all costs. Was the reason distracted driving, or impaired driving, or just a fatal mistake? Recently, I drove across Canada in a Jeep that had a navigational assistance device built in. The device keeps you from hitting other people, keeps you from drifting out of your lane and it can even brake if you don't see a hazard. If tragedies could be cut by even a small percentage, lives could be saved.

I looked at Pepper, and the desire for her to do well and to learn from every call made me realize that there were special people who were in this profession for the right reasons. No matter the outcome today, I could say we did our best. Tomorrow we could try another approach if we faced similar challenges, but at the end of the day we made a difference despite the heavy losses. One of the police officers came over and cleared us to transport the body to the local hospital. The coroner would handle the transport and care from then on. On the way back, it was a silent trip but a respectful trip just the same. Some days there is nothing to say.

At the end of the day we had lost someone's family, someone's daughter, and no matter why the accident occurred, the outcome was a huge loss for many people. When we dropped off the deceased patient, the nurses gave us moral support and provided reassurance to make sure we were okay, having heard what we'd faced today. They all knew the terrible day we'd had. One look inside our bloody unit and they would know we did all we could despite the tragic outcome.

Back at the base, the crew was waiting with coffee and snacks and they all pitched in to strip the unit and restock. There was nothing like a coffee and a snack to help you relax and debrief. We were now about three hours past our normal quitting time and thankfully this shift was finally over. We all sat around after and shared the day's events. The team support was more than appreciated, it was a lifesaver.

The drive home was somewhat relaxing despite the difficult day. I think I was still in shock from the day, but at that point, I was on autopilot and could just drive as a casual driver with no hurry or no expectations. I turned on some music and listened to the songs on my playlist and let the events of the day unfold in my mind. As time passed, I would slowly work through the call in my mind, with the intent of modifying care on a future similar call. That was the art of providing emergency care; we just did our best in the situation we were presented with.

It is often our own critique of events that allows our professional abilities to grow or us to adapt to unique situations. We grow wiser by learning to master difficult situations. New staff are often overwhelmed by certain types of calls. It's no one's fault; it's all about call management. An experienced paramedic can walk in and take over, and in no time a call will be managed, and, in no time, everyone will have a job and the call will be over before you know it. I just prayed that night that my former students had a good mentor to guide them through their initial tragedies. That wasn't too much to pray for, I hoped.

The Right Decisions — My Life in EMS Wisdom Points

- *Be a true hero and accept your wins as well as your losses.*
- *Even with experience, knowledge and wisdom, we can still be wrong.*
- *We aren't meant to be right every time.*
- *We will never always be right, for this is a profession where there is never just one right answer, and, in fact, there can be many possible solutions to a problem.*
- *Never give up.*
- *We can't always win the battle.*
- *We must learn from our mistakes.*
- *It's okay to disagree sometimes.*
- *Not everyone is always right, but you can learn a lot from those with a good track record.*
- *Leroy Jethro Gibbs is a great leader of the* NCIS *team, but even Gibbs can't be expected to do the right thing every time.*
- *Gibbs' Rule 51 clearly states, "Sometimes we are wrong!"*

Chapter 10: Scope of Practice – Our Real Limitations

"Doing What's Right"

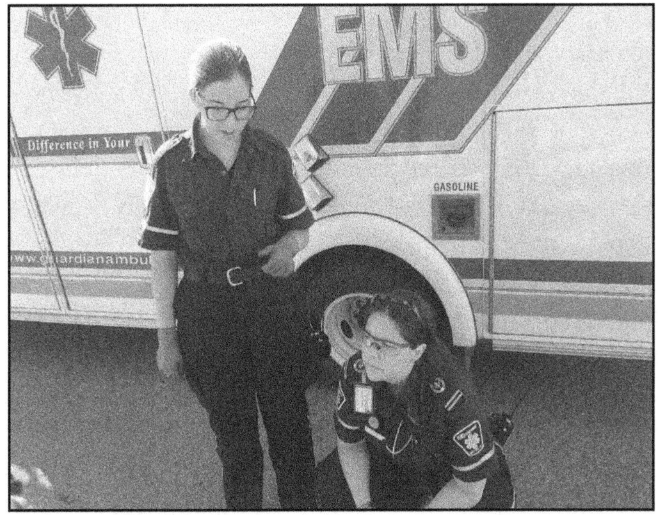

Robyn and Heather: mentor or teacher?

A major problem with our profession is that the scope of practice has evolved at different rates in different locations for a variety of reasons. A scope of practice is essentially defined by the needs of the people who require our services. The needs of the people are different from one province to another. Urban and rural EMS practices are very different as well. When you're ten minutes away from a major hospital versus two hours away, the skill sets required to keep a patient alive are very different.

In rural settings we are always working at trying to get the critical patients stabilized and the critical care centres are trying to always accommodate us when we require a higher level of care. The practitioner must learn how to best care for a patient in any situation.

We may even need different supplies and additional medications. In remote locations, we carry extra medications and supplies as we don't have a place to restock when in isolated locations. But no matter how prepared you think you are, some calls will still stretch your resources to the limits.

A practitioner's skills, and knowledge change in keeping with societal structure. However, regardless of training or scope of practice, you need to know when to utilize certain skills and when to abstain. Having the required training does not automatically give you permission to perform a skill. Having the best-trained or the newest, keenest staff won't do people much good if a patient refuses to be helped. Even as we evolve to be able to better help people, there will always be difficult patients that we must deal with. We must therefore adapt our traditional approach when dealing with such issues as drug abuse, misuse of EMS services and lack of receiving beds in urban centres.

One would not think it possible, but people will refuse care for many reasons, and even if they might suffer without it, it's something we can't do much about. Other people abuse the system by using it as a taxi service. It amazes me when you try everything possible to help people and they still refuse your help, then the next caller is abusing the system. We must always do our best for our patients, regardless of the reasons they call for an ambulance. It is also important to have diversity within the EMS system in order to be able to serve patients in different languages and with different cultural needs. The diversity of our country dictates the unique requirements from the local ambulance services.

The EMS system is made up of many different levels of care providers as set out by provincial and local needs. Often, rural and urban populations are provided with unequal levels of care. Urban areas demand advanced life support (ALS) care within a certain time span while rural areas are lucky to receive basic life support (BLS) care within an hour on a bad day. Often, we see multiple rural services flexed into our urban centres to try to help with increased call volumes. In times of natural disasters or multiple patient traumas, the favour is returned. Examples of this are localized disasters like the Calgary flood, the Slave Lake fire, and the Fort McMurray wildfire where services from multiple provinces pooled their resources to help relieve the added burden on the local system. The outpouring of help was very humbling to see. We are truly a caring nation. Not only did local providers step up, but national and international support was also seen and was very much appreciated.

Levels of care can be different on an individual level, as well; based, for example, on the eagerness of the provider as well as their level of competence. A good practitioner can provide great care, just as a bad practitioner can provide terrible care regardless of having the same theoretical scope of practice. At the end of the day, we simply need to try to do our best regardless of our level of training or who we are treating. If you're nice to others and you care about the people you work with, half the job is already complete.

As an educator, I felt it would be a good time to help laypeople understand our profession a little better in this chapter. We have grown and expanded over the years from a scoop and run "one person" ambulance service in the early 1970s, to a BLS level service in the late 1980s, to providing ALS in many locations in most provinces. Essentially, all initial EMS care is at a basic life support (BLS) level. This level of medical care is used for patients with life-threatening illnesses or injuries until they can be given full medical care at a hospital. It can be provided by trained medical personnel, including emergency medical technicians (now known as primary care paramedics), paramedics, and bystanders qualified in first aid and standard cardiopulmonary resuscitation (CPR).

Just imagine that you are called to the drowning of a child. Irrespective of the level of care, we all approach a case in a similar fashion. The differences lie in what we do after care is initiated and especially after we have resuscitated a patient, if possible. A BLS provider clearly do their best on scene and try to initiate transport as quick as possible. They use the ABCDE approach, which stands for Airway, Breathing, Circulation, Disability and Exposure, covering the basics of care. The "Disability" component is also known as the differential diagnosis stage, which helps us to narrow down the cause of the medical problem to the most likely diagnosis. "Exposure" ensures that we assess the patient thoroughly enough to find any hidden injures.

We then move toward the Advanced Life Support (ALS) level of care. The ALS level provides us with many life-saving protocols and skills that extend our basic life support care to further support circulation with medication and by providing an open airway with adequate ventilation to ensure better oxygenation. After basic care is done, we initiate advanced care. We must still not waste time in transport, but we are expected to spend extra time dispensing medications and applying alternate treatments to boost the ventilation and circulation requirements of a patient who might be unstable. Ideally, we recognize potential complications prior to them occurring and we bypass to the most appropriate care facility.

We always have access to expert assistance from On-Line Medical Control (OLMC) for expert guidance in emergency medical situations in our provincial EMS system. OLMC provides medical oversight in treatment decisions involving patient care in a prehospital setting. A good practitioner knows when to seek expert help and knows when the patient needs that extra care. The biggest obstacle is occasional communication problems in remote locations with low populations and in geographically diverse areas with mountains, hills and valleys where getting a signal can be dicey.

Communicating in dead areas has been one of biggest problems for EMS, fire and police services for years. In EMS, communication failure can break down on multiple levels, from transmission failure of 12-leads in suspected heart attacks, to being unable to reach

OLMC and unable to talk to our dispatchers. There can also be computer failures in the units, portable radio failures, or failure of electronic ePCR tablets. On a bad day, our system of communication fails. Someday, hopefully, we can put our efforts into making a better communication system. Just like everything else, we get what we pay for, and great communication systems are expensive. In the attempt to be fiscally accountable, corners are always cut to save money.

Basic care is started by first responders, who adhere to guidelines or local protocol. First responders are often volunteers, but can be security personal, a police officer, emergency medical responders (EMRs), primary care paramedics (PCPs) or an advanced care paramedics (ACP), all of whom are required to respond to incidents at medical centres or industrial sites. It is very helpful for rural locations to have EMRs, PCPs, and ACPs as volunteer firefighters or on mutual aid teams. They are summoned by either the patient, their coworkers or by Good Samaritans. They are often a part of a team of that is responsible for going immediately to the scene of an emergency event to provide medical assistance. Many industrial sites have a first responder system that can look after medical, fire or site-specific emergencies twenty-four hours a day.

Many areas use volunteers as medical responders when there is not an available ambulance in the community. These responders provide oxygen, first aid and cardiopulmonary resuscitation (CPR) and can use an automatic external defibrillator (AED) when needed. They are considered part of EMS services. As of 2015, first responders, police, firefighters and members of the public are being trained to safely administer Naloxone (Narcan) for suspected opiate overdoses. We have seen a huge call increase in urban locations of people abusing homemade fentanyl products. Recent statistics from the US say about 63,000 people died for the chance to get high in 2016 alone. Hardly worthy of the cost but very deadly just the same. We are all scrambling to avert the death toll but until people realize the risk and the consequences, we are going to keep losing people.

All level of care providers can perform trauma immobilization, fracture care, (including cervical immobilization), and other basic medical care for sick or injured patients in need. In recent years, regulation has relaxed their stance on the use of spine boards and other extrication equipment due to long-term effects seen in people who are immobilized for long periods of time. Just as with all treatments, there are good and bad outcomes from certain procedures. If at all in doubt, you can always call 911 and EMS services will decide on the most appropriate care. Every injury is different, as are patient co-morbidities. Age is a huge factor in the level or type of care a patient will need. There will always be unique situations when we need to consider alternatives in our care or treatments.

Primary care paramedics (PCPs) may also receive additional training to perform certain skills that are normally in the scope of practice of advanced care paramedics (ACPs), such as the application or transmission of a 12-lead EKG to a physician for interpreting sinus rhythms. These results can be captured and sent to anywhere in the world and are regulated provincially (by statute), and locally (by the medical director).

Traditionally, students who want to enter the emergency medical industry must present with a class four driver license, a standard first aid course and the health care provider CPR course. Students can take these courses from many schools and must comply with school's requirements if they want to continue their education. Prior to taking the Emergency Medical Responder (EMR) course, as well as the Primary Care Paramedic (PCP) courses, students must be able to prove that they have a clean criminal record in order to drive or become an attendant or to provide direct patient contact. The EMR course can be taken part-time or full-time and can range from two weeks to three months. The new EMR course will increase up to a sixteen-week course, and will include a more comprehensive program, a driving module, and needed practicum. First responders and EMRs are front-line prehospital care providers in many locations.

Primary care paramedics (PCPs) are the next level. These are the individuals who have been referred to for years as EMTs or ambulance technicians. This modern title affords transferability between all provinces under the National Occupational Competency Profile (NOCP), which is a sort of "free-trade agreement" that allow practitioners to work in other provinces. It also provides a national registration body to help unite practitioners across Canada. PCP courses are full-time and range from three months to two years. The courses are being expanded, and the educational requirements, increased, as the profession grows. As in any profession, there have been some growing pains along the way. Only time and strong leadership will guide our profession forward, along with the collaboration of other allied health professionals. Someday, we will have leaders in the profession with masters and doctorate degrees as practitioners, educators and leaders to enhance the profession across all borders and domains.

The Primary Care Paramedic (PCP) course is the entry level to paramedic practice in most Canadian provinces. The scope of practice of a PCP includes performing semi-automated external defibrillation, cardiac monitoring, and administering oxygen to people with breathing complications, as well as administering a select number of medications. These interventions can make a big difference in many life or death situations. A PCP can start an IV when they need to administer intravenous fluid to patients in hypovolemic shock. They can also provide cardiac monitoring. Cardiac monitoring and EKG interpretation is not an easy skill, but once you master it you won't forget it.

Some services have started implementing non-opiate medications so that primary care paramedics can treat patients who require pain management following provincial protocol. These medications include ketorolac, acetaminophen and ibuprofen. The broader the scope of practice, the more care we can provide in EMS settings. With time, the scope of practice will evolve and someday it will be less restrictive. It is also expected that BLS staff be familiar with

ALS skills as they will often be called on to assist senior staff in emergencies or during our transfers. Good BLS members are often sounding boards for ALS practitioners who have doubts or need some reassurance in their day-to-day calls. Most ALS teams have one BLS and one ALS staff member. Rarely do services have more than one ALS staff member, the exception being services with extra funding or a built-in service requirement from the population they serve.

The word "paramedic" is interchangeable with the terms "EMT Ambulance" and "EMT Paramedic." The modern titles are "primary care paramedic (PCP)" or "advanced care paramedic (ACP)." The highest-level practitioners in the profession are called "critical care paramedics (CCPs)." All are health-care professionals. Most are employed in pre-hospital settings or in out-of-hospital environments when hospitals are not easily accessible. Then work mainly as part of emergency medical services (EMS) to enhance the health care of people in urban, rural and remote locations.

Over the years advanced care paramedics have been able to administer medications classified as "symptom relief" medications, for a variety of emergency medical conditions (including epinephrine, salbutamol, ipratropium bromide, aspirin, nitroglycerine, naloxone, dextrose, thiamine, glucagon, Gravol, Benadryl and nitrous oxide). We have seen our medication drug box hold as many as sixty different medications to as low as sixteen medications over the years.

Historically, the title of "paramedic" has seen misrepresentation and abuse. It is now a legally protected title. I have seen people who have minimal training (e.g. industrial first aid) call themselves paramedics. At the end of the day, in order to use this title, you must meet a standard of training or be certified. Furthermore, you must be able to prove it on a call or while working in patient care to maintain the status. As in any profession, continuing education is required to maintain one's right to practice.

You can call yourself many things but to be able to perform under pressure is the real proof. To add to that, great paramedics are usually caring, dedicated, efficient, and willing to take charge and work long hours to make a difference in others' lives. Sub-par practitioners complain about working too much. The people who are dedicated to making a difference are team players and are good at mentoring, leading and making others see the good on a bad day.

Monitors like our Physio Control LP-12s or LP-15s allow us to diagnose a heart attack. Within minutes of doing a 12-lead EKG, we will know if cardiac involvement is suspected. The machine can analyze the heart and tell us with great accuracy if it's an acute heart attack or not. Sometimes the machine is wrong, but not often. That is why we use our clinical judgment, OLMC and have access to cardiologists or emergency physicians to ensure we are accurate in our assessments. Certain conditions can mimic a heart attack on the monitor, so we need to be just as smart as the machines.

There are other monitors that we use in the EMS industry, such as the Zoll and Philips models, but the Physio Control LP-12s and LP-15s are those most commonly used. We learn to master them as it's part of our profession to master life-saving interventions. When we obtain the 12-leads, we send them to a cardiologist or emergency physician, who can then give us permission to administer clot-busting medication that can reverse the effects of a heart attack. If we can give the clot-busting medications in a timely manner, it can save lives and cardiac muscle. We are often reminded by experts in cardiac care that "time is muscle," and once the muscle is lost, the damage is irreversible.

The fact that we follow protocol and need to use our clinical judgment as well as our experience tells us all the EMS world is complex. Emergency medicine is a dynamic and complex branch of medicine. In some situations, we don't have all the answers, for lack of understanding what the underlying complications are for our patients. Thus, some days we can only do our best with what we have in front of us. I often think of the quote below when we are confronted with complex situations.

**"Sometimes we need to bend the rules to save a life,
but we must not break our moral code, destroy
our ethics or lose our soul along the way."**

—Dale M. Bayliss

Chapter 11: The Right Partner - The Real Challenges

"NoOneWalksAlone"

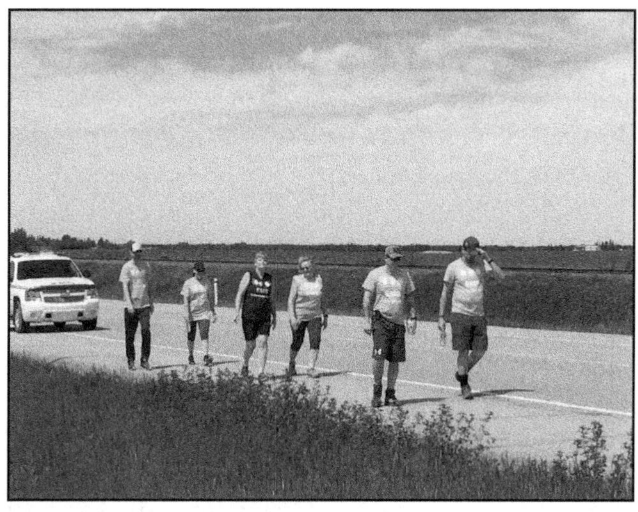

The ultimate team comes from having the right partner. In our line of work, we can't function effectively as a team unless we are committed to the cause. Being a partner on any effective team requires effort, patience and tolerance to make the teamwork. The more synergistically you work together, the better the results will be. Think of it as adding four-wheel drive to good tires compared to trying to drive on poor roads with bald tires. If you have traction and control you can go anywhere you need to go, and it's no different on the job. The right partner is someone who is on your side, and is going to keep you safe, 24/7. This means from the start of your shift to the time you're heading home. A good partner can read your feelings and knows when you could use a coffee and have a break.

Over the years my life has been saved many times by my partner. Know for a fact there are people in the world who will try to cause you harm, if for no other reason than the fact that you are wearing a uniform. We need to watch out for each other. *No One Walks Alone* in today's EMS world.

The one part that is hard to teach is your approach to scenes. We often refer to any given scene as having an outer circle and an inner circle. The inner circle needs to be secure enough for us to perform any treatment. With a partner, you can be aware of what's going on in different directions. This is going ensure that someone is always watching your back and not setting you up for disaster. Often, on scenes, the RCMP flank us when our scene is unsure. You might be busy dealing with an unconscious patient in the living room and not sure who or what lurks beyond in the basement or the bedrooms. When you're busy and you're not able to clear the area, the police will keep you safe.

On your first several calls with your new partner, you're showing them the tricks of the trade, sharing your knowledge and making sure they know what is safe and what is not. Sadly, some days we are so busy we don't get to share the right information as clearly as possible. Most errors or accidents are preventable. The role of the mentor is to groom the new staff. "Get in the ambulance and hang on," I would say. "We are on this next call together. You are now our eyes and ears and you need to watch out for the rest of us. We'll watch out for you, also."

One day, I was working an extra shift with Julie. She will always have a special place in my heart. As my East Coast friends would say, she is the "salt of the earth." We were called to a three-year-old patient who was having seizures and breathing issues. We were very close to the scene, so we had little time to prepare. I said, "Julie, you take airway and monitor. I'll get a SAMPLE and an IV and drugs, as needed." She looked at me and said, "Deal" We had a backup unit coming but it would be ten to twelve minutes away. We had no reason to expect a scene hazard, or problems on scene, but I would soon learn the hard way that that was far from the truth on that day. Sometimes we simply walk into a disaster and we make the best out of it. That's what we do to stay alive on our worst days. No matter what we walk into, we watch out for each other. Today I had one of the toughest ladies watching my back and she had me watching hers. That's all that mattered.

As we pulled up to the place, I started to get a bad feeling. I said to Julie, "Watch out, my lady. We might be in trouble." I just had this eerie feeling. That same feeling had saved my life a few times in the past. We grabbed our kits and walked to the apartment door. We knocked but got no response. I tried the door and it opened. It was the right address and I had never been here before, so I had no past knowledge of what to expect. As we stepped in, I yelled "Ambulance! We're here to help!" The place was a mess and we heard some voices in the back room. I reached for my radio mic and was ready to call for help. We just kept walking ahead and looking for a child that needed our help. There had to be a child here, someplace.

In seconds, with our kits at our sides, we entered the first bedroom we came to, where we both saw a toddler in serious trouble. We set our kits down and made a dash for the kid lying on the floor in front of us. He was bleeding from the side of his head, and it looked as if he had been bleeding for a long time. The smaller the child, the less reserve of blood they have, so this was likely life-threatening bleeding. Julie was right at my side. She looked at me and nodded that she was okay, as this was one of her first serious calls. She was grabbing some trauma dressing while I put pressure on the laceration with my gloved hand. The situation was less than ideal. We should likely not have been there, but we were and that was the scary part of working EMS. Today we had walked into serious trouble. More trouble was soon to come.

I was wondering where the parents or guardians were, when from another room a lady staggered into view. She was stumbling, likely impaired, and looked to have been assaulted recently as well. A man followed her, and he started yelling at us. He was aggressively coming right at us. We were in trouble. I pushed the panic button on the portable radio and I said to Julie, "Save the kid." I quickly turned my back on my partner to face on of my biggest challenges yet: a giant of a man charging at us. I'd intended to try to talk to him and reason with him. Usually that worked, but it was apparent that it wasn't going to work this time. The only thing I knew for sure was that we were going to save this kid. But we were also going to need to get the heck out of here, right now! That's when I knew in my heart that it was too late to avoid getting hurt ourselves.

The guy kept coming at me and he had something in his hand; out of the corner of my eye, I could see it was a weapon of some sort. I didn't take my eyes off his as I had to know his intent and respond as required. I wished I knew what it was that he held in his hand, but he was coming too fast, and he was way too close. My options were simple: we were in life-threatening danger. I dropped him with a flying football tackle and pinned him, as I fought to grab the arm holding the weapon. Then at least he couldn't hurt anyone. Julie, I knew, would do her part for the child to try to stop the bleeding. Her next course of action would be to retreat with the child in her arms and hopefully with me at her side. I had a sudden flashback to the 1991 movie *Backdraft* when firefighter Stephen McCaffrey says to his partner, "You go, we go!" I just needed a way to make it happen—and sooner than later was better for all of us. Today, we needed help. We were both praying, and I was sure it was coming in the next minute.

I struggled to free what was in his hand and realized it was an old metal iron. I was trying to get control of the hand with the weapon, but I could not get it free from his hand. This was not what I expected to be doing today, but regardless we were here, and this had to stop right now. I could only hold him for so long and then what else could I do? Out of the corner of my eye, I could see the intoxicated female staggering toward me and yelling at me.

I had to make a decision and it was simple: we had to get out *now*. We would fight our way out with Julie holding the kid. Today was definitely not a "stay and play" day; today was good day to just run.

Miraculously, two rapidly moving police officers with weapons drawn suddenly burst through the apartment door. I was never more thankful to see our police backup. No matter how much they pay any police officer, it never could compensate them enough for the dangers they respond to daily. One of them subdued and controlled the aggressive female, who was about to strike me or her husband/boyfriend, I wasn't sure. I didn't think it mattered as I was in the middle, so I'd be hit anyways. The other officer must have realized there was a weapon and he didn't waste a second helping me. Two firefighters followed the officers in, and they immediately scooped up Julie and the child and were out of the apartment just as quickly with the kits in tow. They all knew what to do without a single word being spoken. It was a good idea to retreat. "Save the ones you can," is not a bad motto for any situation.

Thank God for backup. It was like getting a gold medal for winning a life-saving race. For years we have worked together with police and fire, and today it was as if we had rehearsed the scenario to a T, even if I can't think of this scenario ever being practiced. This was a tactical hostage and police scenario, only it was it all too real. We could never dream this one up and I had participated in many practice scenarios over the years. I was happy to have my bulletproof vest on; it blunted the hits to my chest tonight, and I was just thankful it was not being tested by a knife or a bullet. Getting stabbed or shot was not on my list of things to try before I retired.

I knew that alarms would be ringing in the dispatch centre and every unit working that day would have heard our distress call. It would be very stressful for our co-workers. The poor dispatchers on the other end of the radio would be panicking. They would have heard nothing but silence after they radioed us, as we hadn't had a chance to return their calls. But sometimes we couldn't prevent communication failures.

More police stormed in and took over the bad guy's immediate care. I extricated myself from him as fast as possible and scrambled out of the room. I knew Julie needed me, and the little boy needed me even more right now. Julie would be worried about me for that was who she was, but she also knew I was tough and had some scars to prove it. I had almost made it to the door when my vision started to play tricks on me. I thought to myself, "Not today." It had happened to me a few times before but very seldom, mostly after hitting my head too hard. Now was not a good time to pass out.

Suddenly, the dizziness hit me. Another firefighter noticed I was having trouble, grabbed my arm and helped me stay on my feet. It's scary how fast your brain can become off-balance. In a few seconds, I felt okay, and we gathered up the remaining kits and made off to the unit. It was only then that I realized that I had been in one very dangerous battle. Luckily, he hadn't been able to get a good swing at me. I had kept the iron from being used and didn't think I was even hurt. I had no signs of bleeding, and nothing was broken. It was nothing serious, even if I had been struck a few times with his fist. Being hit is sometimes a good wake-up call, anyway. It gets the adrenalin pumping in a hurry.

We were not supposed to have physical battles on the job, but it happened nonetheless. I'd much rather be hit or hurt than let someone hurt my partner. My many years of dealing with aggressive people and helping save people paid off today, as I knew many ways to protect myself and how to block my attacker's hits and kicks. The rule was simple: if you got into a battle for your life, you needed to win, and you needed to stay alive at all costs. The safety of everyone on the team is paramount to our job. On this day we got out of a bad situation in the best condition we could hope for.

I jumped into the back of the unit and saw a RCMP officer helping Julie with the child on the stretcher. I would have bet he had past emergency medical training as I watched him help my partner. They were working on airway management by suctioning secretions and blood to clear the child's small airway and applying oxygen. I could see the worry in Julie's eyes. Rapidly, the bleeding was controlled, the airway was cleared, and supplemental oxygen flowed at a high rate to accommodate for any hypoxia prior to our arrival. We were simply giving supplemental oxygen. Thankfully, the child began breathing better after the airway was cleared, which was very good to see. Dispatch was frantically calling us, but neither of us had replied because our hands had been busy. Thank God our distress buttons worked. They were responsible for sending police, fire and additional EMS units our way. Every crew for hundreds of miles would know we were in trouble, and anyone who was close could come to our rescue if they were dispatched. Even if they were not, they might deviate in our direction just in case.

When Julie and I were both safe, I finally acknowledged the dispatcher, letting them know that we were safe, but that we had "run into a little trouble." The police had secured the scene and two people were in custody. We could explain that part later. I asked for help from the PICU, Critical Care and the OLMC right away. They would simply conference them all in. I set my phone by the LP-15 and we kept working. We could hear sirens coming from different directions to our rescue still. That was real music to my ears.

We both looked at each other and smiled. I simply said, "That was close," to which Julie nodded and said, "Maybe a little too close." Overall, we had been lucky despite my little wrestling match. I could have used Rocky or even Rambo for a few seconds in the apartment, but we made it through just the same. When this call was done we were going to take an extra-long break. Then maybe my heart rate and my BP would normalize.

We had our hands full, even if our patient was a lot smaller than our regular trauma patients. We all hated sick and injured kid calls the most, I would say. Over the years, the Pediatric Advanced Life Support (PALS) courses had taught us some valuable tricks to help sick and injured children. It would be my partner's first such call, but she was truly gifted, and she would follow my lead. We also had backup coming and they would be arriving soon.

Today, we had no air support to transport, so we planned to bypass, meet the extra ALS help on the way, and then continue to the pediatric trauma centre. I inserted an IV and Julie kept working with the police officer, who was helping as well to apply monitors, assess vitals and update the other people listening on the radio. A quick primary and secondary survey told us that the child was unconscious and had a closed head injury, a compromised airway likely with facial fractures, and multiple new and old bruises to his little body. Julie filled me in on what she knew and had seen. She had on artificial airway and was setting up to start assisting with ventilation. I had not seen a case of child abuse as bad as this in years. Of all the calls we get, they have to be some of the worst.

A firefighter, also a PCP, was elected to be our driver today by the fire captain on scene. The instructions to my driver, even if they were not really needed for this transfer, were clear and easy. "Easy on the corners and giv'er on the straightaways." He laughed at me and said, "Roger, Captain." He was no rookie. Today our speed was not going to be debated. We needed a PICU team and a neurosurgeon or this little one would not survive. In no time we were off with the police officer who was helping us in back. As we left the scene, we saw the other backup unit heading toward us on the open highway. We pulled over and picked up the extra help. Then we took off like a rocket one more time. It was an ALS crew from another service that I had not worked with before, but they immediately jumped in and went to work. We were a team. Throughout the transfer, we kept the little man stable. Even with such tragic injuries, he was a real fighter.

On route, we debated doing an advanced airway but ended up just using an alternate airway, which worked for now. The KING airway was working despite my reluctance to use them. We knew the anesthesiologist and the pediatrician would insert an advanced airway, but so far, we'd had no trouble, so we just made do with what we had. The patient's SpO2 and CO2 were within normal range, so we were happy to wait. We got everything set up for an advanced airway and had the medications ready, watched the monitors and kept reassessing, and thankfully we arrived with a stable but critical child.

The pediatric trauma team took over making the care decisions and in no time were off to the CT scanner with the pediatrician and neurosurgeon at the little one's side. Our end goal was to keep him alive and now it was the critical care staff and PICU staff that would make the difference. The child's fate was now out of our hands.

We went to our unit and sat down for a much-needed break and debrief. Our debriefing started and finished in the ambulance bay with our police officer, the backup crew and our firefighter driver. One of the security staff and another crew member got us coffee. A few extra crew started cleaning and stocking our unit. I took a moment to call and thank the dispatcher, and to explain briefly what had happened. We would still need to provide statements to the police and complete our ePCR, but I could work on that on the way back to our base. We all needed time to reflect on the call and talk about the events. We would do a formal debriefing in the next few days. Right now, we needed to just breathe and take in the fact that we were safe.

After we got back to base, our shift was technically not over, but our supervisor ended our shift anyway. We had both seen and done enough for one day. A quick trip to the police station to file our statements followed, and the whole shift was now a blur. I thought back to what occurred, and I still could not comprehend it all. Thinking about what we could have changed or done differently is always easier done retrospectively. The only thing we could have done differently was maybe back out and let the police go in first, but then what about the bleeding child? I'd like to think that we learned that anything is possible, and no matter what, we need to stick together and communicate in stressful situations. Also, it helps to have a game plan. As I've learned the hard way over the years, it's important to always have a backup plan as well. When that fails, make the best out of what you have left. Just ensure that you and your partner are safe.

Essential Requirements for Paramedics:
Must be dedicated, sincere, caring, honest, and willing to be lifelong learners.

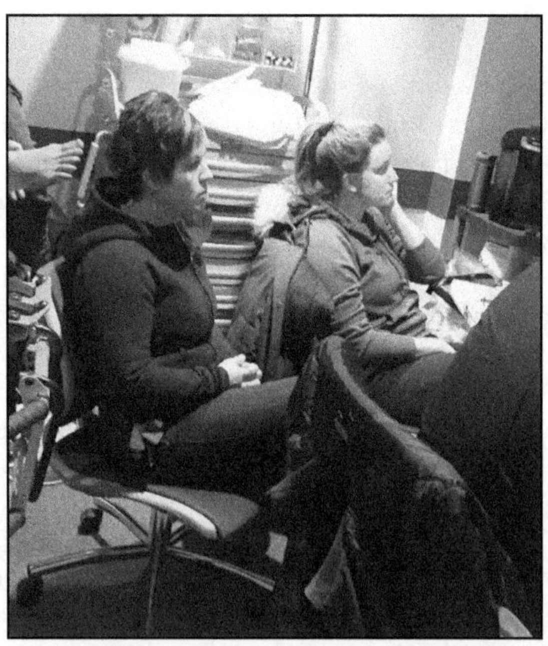

My motto: You can never be taught too much. Training is mandatory to get it right – we need to practice until we can't fail.

Chapter 12: Educational Requirements to Save a Life

"Knowing Enough to Get By"

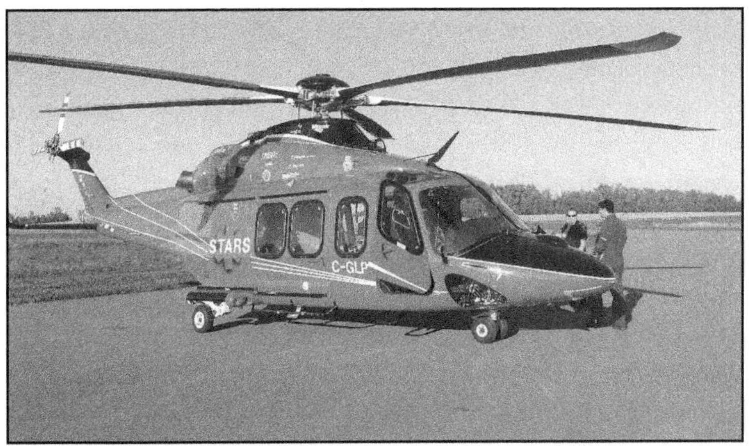

One aspect of emergency medicine is that you can't prepare for complex cases that have abnormal presentations. The calls that have stumped me the most are the ones that have unusual or strange presentations. The more you know about emergency medicine, the more you will appreciate a good place to visit when you're sick or injured. From pain control, to emergency surgery on the trauma room stretcher, to the practice of internal medicine, emergency medicine is much more complex than it seems. When new students look at us for guidance on what they need to learn, it makes me appreciate more what I've likely forgotten.

One day shift started with a figurative bang: two serious calls right after each other. We had just cleaned up after a call and we were responding to another. Salt was doing her best to be an efficient and safe driver, but today, people on the roads were not paying attention to their driving or merely ignoring the people around them. I could hear her mumbling words that I can't repeat after we were cut off at two separate locations. Pepper was my partner, as I was her mentor today. It was my job to sit back and give her guidance while she ran the show. This was an easy thing for some but a hard task for me.

I like to teach, but sometimes, you need to be silent and let junior staff figure things out on their own. It's not being rude, it's just part of letting people find their own way to manage calls. I was just there for backup if the call turned out to be complex, or if something bad happened. We were paged for a pediatric seizure and were not wasting any time. I hate sick and injured pediatric calls for a good reason. Today, having an extra staff member on the call was a big relief. There are many days that having an extra person on hand would have been magical. My worst call was doing one-man CPR in the back of an ambulance while trying to ventilate, start an IV and give adrenalin. My driver was a volunteer and I was simply happy for him to drive. That would have been a great day for backup or an extra set of hands, but it was not available. Some days we needed to "scoop and run" and that was one of those days.

Dispatch information said a parent had called in the emergency, stating it was a seizure. The caller must have been in the medical field, as she was very helpful to the dispatcher and gave a SAMPLE history, which they relayed to us. It was a thirteen-year-old male having a first-time seizure. On our arrival, the seizure was over, and the patient appeared to be sleeping, but something looked wrong as he lay on the couch in the living room. Moreover, something sounded wrong as we walked into the room. We all heard the snoring respirations at the doorway and quickly picked up the pace. I knew my partners would be great, but I quickly paged for a backup unit, just in case, and let the dispatcher know we were in trouble. They could then get us extra assistance when the time was appropriate. We had an unstable pediatric patient with some very serious, but unknown, conditions that were more than likely to make this situation worse by the second.

Pepper took over the airway care and started asking for airway and breathing adjuncts as she quickly assessed the boy. She quickly performed a modified jaw-thrust maneuver as Salt passed her what she needed. I applied the monitor, as well as started to get additional history from the parents. After a few seconds we all heard what we expected to hear. We all knew there had to be a reason for this event. The parents informed us that the boy had been riding his bike and crashed after hitting a curb. He'd had his helmet on, and the helmet had cracked. That told us that there had been enough impact to cause a head injury. The boy had come home after the crash and had gotten sleepy. The parents had no idea he had a serious head injury.

Salt finished the quick primary and secondary surveys after the ventilations improved. Pepper stayed with the airway care. All we could find was a hematoma on the side of the head and some swelling to the frontal area as well. I asked our dispatcher to launch STARS and asked if they could send a doctor as well. We considered our transport times and a small hospital was close; we needed to go there first, and they could meet us in the emergency room. This way, we would have a local physician to help us with treatments and access to extra medications (such as mannitol), if needed. Today was not a day to waste time.

The next decision was what to do about the airway. This was one time where oxygenation and ventilation could save a life or better yet save a brain. Pepper was doing a great job of ventilating to ensure that the end-tidal CO2 was in a safe range, but it needed to be perfect. The heart rate was trending downward, and the BP was trending up, and it was imperative to ensure we did our jobs perfectly to save this child's life. One wrong step or one wrong dose of medication could result in a disaster. I weighed the pros and cons of transporting with the airway as it was versus performing an advanced airway. I considered many past intubations—what went right and what went wrong—and I weighed the odds in a few seconds. We needed to just make it happen right now.

It was supposed to be Pepper's call, but today experience and expertise was needed, and there was no time to debate the options. I said, "Let's tube him right now." The backup crew had just come in the door and they had a good idea we were in trouble. John walked up to me and said, "What do you need my friend?" I had the plan already in my head. We quickly discussed the steps that needed to be done and, like magic, the child was being prepared for an advanced airway. We were providing high-flow oxygen through nasal prongs and assisting the breathing with our BVM. Greg, our supervisor, was preparing the medications needed while another staff member was preparing the intubation tubes. Another member grabbed a second suction device just in case. You could never be too careful. When you're using medications to secure an airway, you're making the patient's breathing and ventilation rate stop or be ineffective. Ideally, the best suction was in the hospital, but today we would make it work with our portable suction.

The medications were double-checked to make sure we had the right concentrations, the right dosages, and that they were in the right order to administer as they were needed. It was like clockwork. They all had to be given in the right order, with the right timing to ensure they were flushed in carefully with normal saline flushes, but not too quickly as we could cause hypotension. An extra IV was inserted in case it might be needed if the primary IV site blew or caused other untoward effects. There was no room for errors or failures, for we only had one chance, and if we caused side effects, we could have a terrible outcome. All our years of experience, of taking extra courses, had given us the knowledge, wisdom and confidence to make the right decisions. Every intubation we had performed over the years had given us the confidence to make the right decision when it was needed the most.

One mistake could kill the boy or make him an organ donor. That was the best-case scenario, if we were lucky. We had all seen tragedies involving children and to realize we could change the outcome from life to death made the scenario all too real. Some days you can get so scared you don't do anything on the ALS side and BLS is often not enough to prevent the inevitable tragedies. But in saying that, if we caused the child to have a hypoxic brain from not being able to intubate, we weren't doing anyone any good. The golden rule was to "do no harm" to our patients, and that was especially true when it came to kids.

A quick conference with a critical care physician, the OLMC and the local ER doctor ensued. The STARS team was coming, and they would bring a neurosurgeon or pediatrician on board. They were already on the roof of the trauma hospital, so they had access to resources we would never have. I could see the crew members positioning the child with his head slightly raised to help decrease the cerebral edema, and a cervical collar was applied as a safety precaution in case of a spinal injury. As we prepared the patient, we also prepared the parents. I was nominated as the team leader. Firefighters showed up to help and brought us our scoop, the stretcher and extra supplies.

The local RCMP arrived and they quickly took over helping with the parents and would get the family support from Victim Services, as well. It's never a bad idea to involve the police right away, as some pediatric cases can be suspicious. The police ensure we are safe, as well. You never know when the scene dynamics can change and there is no such thing as a "normal" call, so being prepared for the worst is always advisable. This scene was very busy but controlled. You could feel the love in the air. Not one person was arrogant or condescending. We were a team and today we had to be the best team in the world. In no time, we had all the local EMS resources working together to help save a life. That is a very satisfying feeling.

In mere minutes, an artificial airway was in place, secured, checked and rechecked, ensuring it was exactly in the right spot. Pepper took over the BVM care and watching the monitor like it was her lifeline. Salt ensured the child was immobilized and that we were not missing anything. The second crew prepared extra medications. The child was stabilized and ready for transport in record time. STARS was on route and would be ready to assist after they arrived at the local ER. The ER staff were ready and waiting for us as well.

Our firefighters volunteered to drive us and helped get the patient moved to the unit. As soon as we got into the unit and the doors were closed, I said, "Pepper, it's your call now. I'll take over the BVM and you are now my boss." She smiled and took over the call. She was now in charge of two very experienced paramedics and the extra PCPs; the show was now hers. I was so proud of her. In seconds, she had us all organized and she stepped back to assess the whole situation. The skill of mastering a situation is an art in itself. The closer you are to the patient, the less you can see as the leader, so by her mentally detaching herself and being able to see the monitor, the IVs, the whole scene from a step back, she could make informed decisions.

The transport was unremarkable, yet impressive. Pepper had control and I could watch the show unfold. We were off the scene with a convoy of EMS vehicles. The parents were following right behind us with the police and the backup unit, as well as the fire crews, following. In front of us, local police made sure we were given the right of way as we proceeded through intersections carefully. Salt was too busy to notice but the drivers never got in our way this time.

On arrival, we were met in the ambulance bay by the local emergency physician. She was a brilliant doctor and knew exactly what she needed to do to save a life. We also had the local on-call anesthesiologist present in case we had airway complications. They were thinking ahead. The only thing we hadn't done was an oral gastric tube, but that, as well as a quick chest X-ray, could be done after the CT scan was completed. Today that was the priority. The anesthesiologist took over the airway, and we were off to the scanner. The emergency nurses took over patient care. The child was now their sole responsibility.

Thankfully, they had a CT scanner ready and waiting for us. A CT scan, short for a "computed tomography" scan, produces computer-processed readings of multiple X-ray measurements taken from consecutive sections of an affected body part to produce a series of images that look like slices. As the radiologist or trained physician reviews the CT results, they can see the normal and abnormal scans in seconds. They can even enhance pictures with special contrast dye, but today that wasn't needed. The scan showed a small skull fracture with a nasty hematoma below the surface.

That hematoma was the big problem. It would be putting pressure on the brain and would be the cause of the seizure, as well as the reason the child was unconscious. I could see the bag of mannitol make its way to the CT scanner. The nurse had a filter in place in seconds and as soon as the order was present, it could be started. Hypertonic saline is used in some cases and may help lessen the cerebral swelling, but the decision to use it or not was for the hospital staff to decide and not for us. STARS arrived to bring the child to a hospital with neurosurgery capabilities, and the excitement was over.

There were many complex decisions to be made that day. A dose of TXA (tranexamic acid) can be given to lessen cerebral bleeding if used within three hours of the injury, and there was also the question of optimal head positioning as well as the question of proper ventilation rates. These debates would be carried out by the neurosurgeon, pediatrician, emergency physician, and the radiologist. Everything we do has consequences and affects the big picture, which leads to survival rates and mortality rates of our patients. No matter how much we learn, we still fall short in the critical care areas for many reasons.

As emergency care providers, we do our best, but we are constantly reminded that medicine is always evolving. Researchers are constantly reviewing our patient care results as well as participating in retroactive studies to help evolve the fields of medicine. We often see specialists not agreeing on treatment options for the simple fact that all parts of medicine and surgical interventions are changing as the profession progresses. If you look at the role of a paramedic over the last three generations, there have been so many changes and alterations to our practice. The medications, treatment options, and diagnostic options have all expanded faster than many of us can keep up.

The art of teaching our EMS students has been altered due to big changes in simulation technology. Some feel simulation can take away the need for an extended practicum. I think it can be helpful but nothing beats real calls when it comes to experience. At the end of a student's practical component, they need to master the art of patient care. The real learning starts the first day of employment. If new staff can be mentored and supported, they will soon master the art of being a practitioner.

Following our arrival to the local ER, the child went straight to the scanner which displayed the suspicious lesion. We all sat and discussed the case as we cleaned the unit and restocked the kits. The reality is, nothing but experience can prepare us for the calls we attend. Teamwork is the real key to being part of the EMS profession. The stronger the team, the more efficient we are as a prehospital care team. From students to experienced providers, we all make our team better.

The more education we achieve throughout our career, the more we expand our ability to be better practitioners. Someday, I hope that staff will be required to continually expand their education to be true masters of our profession. The minimal level to gain entry to our profession needs to be increased to ensure our profession does not become extinct. I will leave it to my students and my fellow co-workers to ensure our profession survives. I know Salt and Pepper won't let me down. I believe they will mentor me someday, and that's just fine.

Chapter 13: Facing the Bad

"Fighting the Worst of the Worst Outcomes"

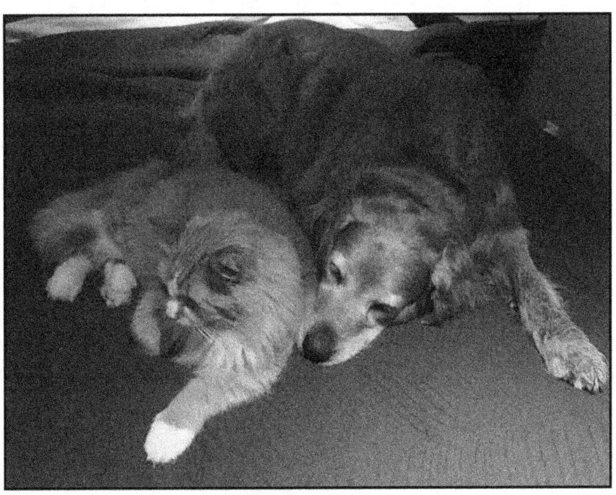

In Emergency Medical Services, we often refer to calls as "good" or "bad." Good calls are the easy ones where a patient is not really that sick. These calls are adrenalin rushes for the staff. We rush to a call, but on arrival, it's not as bad as expected. A patent may need an ambulance, but their condition is not life-threatening. A "bad" call is when someone's life is on the line. It might be an airway, breathing, or circulation emergency, or anything else that alters the level of a patient's consciousness. Once it becomes a life-threatening call, we become much more alert and vigilant with regard to reversing the threat. We are constantly looking for additional problems or assessing unknown conditions and praying the outcome is improved. We apply basic life support (BLS) or advanced life support (ALS) skills as they are needed, and we hope for the best. On a good day, we have a positive outcome. Our interventions help to improve the situation. Not all days are good. Some days just keeps spiraling downwards.

Sometimes, our magic fails to work. On bad days our healing touch is ineffective. Then we resort to applying anything or everything we know to intervene. We face the challenge with determination and attack the life threats with vengeance. We are poor losers. We don't easily admit defeat, for it's not who we are. Sadly, on certain calls we are doomed from the start, and no matter our interventions or our wisdom we will lose the battle to save a life. Everything we try fails and the patient continues to deteriorate.

On our bad days we perform our interventions and administer medications not knowing if they will work and if the patient is going to improve or continue to deteriorate. For example, we may be dispatched for a car accident resulting in a traumatic injury. When we arrive on scene, we assess and triage our patient, and attempt to manage the call in a logical and methodical manner. But despite our interventions, the patient's condition continues to deteriorate. As the call progresses, the patient becomes unresponsive and then suffers a cardiac arrest. We started the call on a high but that rapidly deteriorates to a low, when we realize we have no other option but to stop our resuscitation efforts.

Bad calls are unpredictable, and they will come whether we are ready for them or not. It's possible to prepare for a disaster or emergency by having a plan and making sure resources are available, but you can't easily plan for a bad day. We can learn how to react to specific situations as a team, which will help in the short term. We can learn how to process a scene and figure out an emergency exit plan, if needed, but there is no magical solution to a bad situation.

As we so often face death and destruction, it can be easy to lose sight of the good outcomes amongst all the bad. The following call was one of those times.

Salt, Pepper and I were at Tim Hortons, recharging with a coffee. There was nothing like a coffee with friends. The staff at Timmy's treated me very special. Once they heard my voice at the drive-through window, they knew it was me and they knew my order. I always ordered for my puppies first. Cheese tea biscuits were their favourite.

Both Salt and Pepper were ready to be paramedic students. They would give the teachers a run for their money. Both would challenge the level of learning and exceed the basic requirements and make sure they were well rounded at the end of the program. They were registered in the course, and they would soon be my students again.

We had a good team that day. Our BLS backup crew were Connor and Julie. They were also past students of mine but today they were on a transfer, so we couldn't bug them over a coffee. We were "Alpha One" and they were "Tango Three." We were on together for the next forty-six hours of a forty-eight-hour shift, so it would go by fast.

The morning was unremarkable. We got the unit checks done. The unit was full of fuel, every required piece of equipment was checked and accounted for, the LP-15 was fully charged, and our electric stretcher was charged and ready. We had just taken a seat at Timmy's when we were toned out. The dispatch message said it was a shooting. We had been dispatched for a Staged Event, meaning that the police would be involved, and until they cleared the scene of threats or harm, we were not allowed to arrive on scene at all.

We grabbed our coffee and were off—"Code 4"—which meant lights and sirens. We would waste no time. I was driving. I was terrible at the CAD (computer-aided dispatch) system. I was past my expiration date when it came to technology updates. I had some suggestions to make the system better, but they would not go very far in our current system. I just smiled and nodded when we had system failures due to technological failures. It had been somebody's great idea to take away our ability to see if we had other units coming. We were often left in the dark, which in the rural EMS system is dangerous and not helpful to the crews that are in electronic darkness. Isolation does not contribute to a team approach when it comes to co-responders knowing when and where you need help.

On route, we were told that the shooting had occurred at the local trailer park. RCMP would secure the scene and we would stage and enter only when they had a secure area. They could defend themselves and we could not. We were not bullet-resistant, even if some days we felt like we were. We could see the area and knew the best way in and the fastest way out. As we approached the scene, we could see three RCMP vehicles surrounding the trailer, from all possible directions. In seconds the police were out of their trucks, running to seek cover for themselves and covering each other in case it was a setup, or not what it was called in as. They would not be taken by surprise, for police services around the world had learned important lessons from past shootings. They would also have additional backup on the way. You could never be too safe. We would their backup for now or help them if something terrible went down. There is nothing worse than seeing one your own being shot, but it is part of the job. Nobody is immune to violence.

Within two minutes of being staged, we were given clearance to go in. Salt and Pepper took the lead. I brought up the rear. Salt had the LP-15 monitor, Pepper the ALS airway kit, and I brought up the rear with the trauma bag. We were ready for almost anything. As Salt and Pepper entered, they were confronted by a very traumatic scene. The presentation was a man in his mid-fifties with a non-salvageable head injury from a high-powered rifle lying in the middle of the living room floor. A RCMP member was consoling the man's partner, who immediately became our sole surviving patient. The weapon was secured, and we were all going to be safe.

We had a plan of attack, even if we never said a single word. Pepper immediately took over the role of grief worker and approached the family member. Salt and I quickly applied the monitor to confirm our initial impression. A quick-thinking officer took a picture of the scene to record its initial presentation. The rifle was still across the man's chest and I carefully helped the closest police member remove and then secure it. The man was in asystole and apneic. A pool of blood surrounded him on the floor and part of his cranium and brain was splattered on the wall. I quickly made sure Salt was okay, as this was her first bad call that I was aware of. Salt silently gave me the thumbs-up sign with a few tears noticeable on her cheeks, as Pepper knelt in front of the grief-stricken woman.

We always try to help our patients if it is possible, but some days, it is over the second they pull the trigger. The only hope now was that the decedent could become a transplant donor. That would be the only good that could come out of the devastation. Sadly, this was often the case following bad motorbike and quad accidents, as well. The brain is so delicate, complex and mostly unforgiving of injury. The head is not made to be a baseball. The brain suffers devastating initial injury from the projectile—the smash to the head—followed by the devastating coup/contra-coup injury with the brain being smashed back and forth.

The projectile itself is the structural component of injury, but there is also the blast effect and the resulting tertiary effect from the swelling and tearing of surrounding tissues. Immediately after the overt damage, it is made worse by the body's malfunctioning systems, which increase the buildup of CO2 and waste-causing hypoxia. This further increases the insult to the brain, causing the brain stem to malfunction. Add to that a lack of adequate breathing followed by secondary injury from lack of circulation, as well as anoxia, and hope is lost within minutes after any significant severe head injury. Looking back, I think most of these patients die within the first few minutes.

The scene was quickly secured, and additional officers arrived, along with "Tango Three," as our backup. Connor and Julie quietly slipped around the police officer at the front door and made sure we were okay. We called dispatch to notify them that we would be sending one patient requiring grief counselling and that the initial patient was deceased. I asked the BLS crew to grab a stretcher to transport from "Tango One" with Pepper's assistance, while Salt and I wrote this one up. We assisted them to the door and then assisted Pepper with getting the family member out of this horrific mess. It was easier to split our crews to ensure we accomplished all goals and provided emotional and peer support to co-workers at the same time.

You can never rush the grief process, but eventually, we all knew there would be an appropriate time to get going. The family member's hands and her clothes were covered in blood, but that was the least of our worries. Julie placed a blanket around her and led her outside, strapping her to the stretcher. Her initial vital signs were taken, and she would be given some sedation prior to transport, if needed. Pepper asked if I could give her something and I was more than happy to accommodate.

Once in the unit we quickly administered a sedative and she would be monitored her on our way to the local ER. That day we couldn't save the patient who ended his life prematurely, but we could support his partner and ensure the best possible outcome for her. With the proper grief counselling and long-term support, she would get past this day, but not easily.

After they left the scene, we completed the ePCR and ensured that our documentation was as accurate as possible. The police would ensure that the scene was secured and let the investigation unfold to conclude this case. It's disturbing to work around bodies after such tragedies, knowing that, just minutes before the event they were alive. In some ways, they were still there, even if their life was over. It's strange how you can feel the presence of life or the coldness of death. It's one thing you never get accustomed to, and I think that is a good thing.

The newest staff are the ones we need to protect the most, but we all suffer the consequences of seeing the repeated death and destruction of people from both accidental and intentional self-harm. The hardest thing is seeing the kids, the innocent bystanders in bad situations. They are the ones who are left to feel the hurt and pain of possibly the worst day of their life. One song that says it all too well is by Sequoyah Rain and titled "The Angel." So many parts of the song echo my past experiences working in EMS. Please download it and give it some thought. Don't dwell on it but remember that everyone has bad days. That's when we need each other the most.

"The Angel" by Sequoyah Rain

The Angel of Death came again today
Took some poor soul's life away
I raced as fast as I could to get there by his side
But that Angel's swept him away
Yes, that Angel swept him away

Chorus

And I fly down the highway
Got no time to kill
Only the Lord knows if we'll win
It's a race against the clock
The golden hour's all he's got
There's a desperation in the cool night of wind
Can't let that Angel win again.

Verse

Stop to grab a quick bite to eat
And once again they're calling me
She's tired of life and she took some pills
Her husband left, and her momma died
There is no one left to stand by her side
Its lonely nights leave a bitter chill
And no one else knows how she feels

Chorus

And I fly down the highway
Got no time to kill
Only the Lord knows if we'll win
It's a race against the clock
The golden hour's all he's got
There's a desperation in the cool night of wind
Can't let that Angel win again

Verse

Woke up at two o'clock
Can't stop now, don't have time to walk
She ran her car off of a bridge
I wipe the tears out of her eyes
As she tells her baby goodbye
Another young soul was lost today
Why did she have die this way?

Chorus

And I fly down the highway
Got no time to kill
Only the Lord knows if we'll win
It's a race against the clock
The golden hour's all he's got
There's a desperation in the cool night of wind
Can't let that Angel win again
The Angel of Death came again today
Took some poor soul's life away

This song talks about a difficult subject covering a lot of personal ground for EMS professionals. We never know when we start our shift what will happen over the next hours, or the impact we will have on others' lives. We may all respond as individuals, but at the end of the day we are a team. The role of the team after a call like this one is to ensure we all respond as a team, work as a team and leave as a team. No one should be left out from the team mentally, emotionally or spiritually. As we leave the scenes of disasters, we need to look after each other. We never know how much these types of call will affect us. In the days following a crisis like the one I just described, we need to do our buddy checks to ensure our co-workers are okay.

Some days, we may look okay, but we can be in shock ourselves. Often, it's due to the cumulative effects of calls, to being tired, or to similar calls in the past that make the present call all too real, perhaps triggering a flashback. Let's not allow one of our co-workers to become a statistic. Let's all get home safely. Let's all stay safe for many years to come. With time, education and team effort, we can overcome any hurdle. At the end of a call, during a call and anytime afterwards, *No One Walks Alone* on my crew or among my friends.

We Will Never Forget

September 11/ 2001

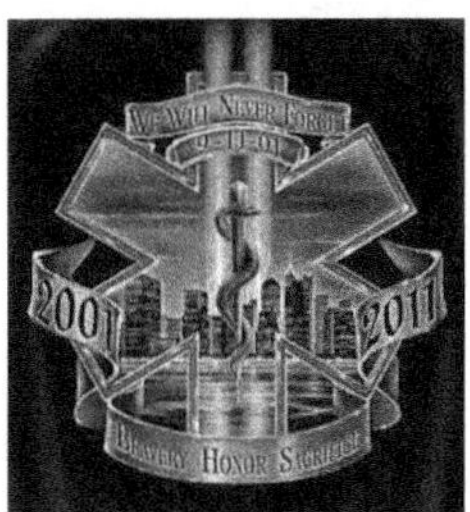

Total lost: 412 EMS Workers

- ***8 Emergency Medical Technicians and Paramedics***
- ***343 Firefighters***
- ***72 Law Enforcement Officers***
- ***Total Lost that one day was 2977 souls, plus many more injured, and those who died after that day due the side-effects of their involvement.***

Chapter 14: Fighting with the Good

"Using the Trauma Team Mentality"

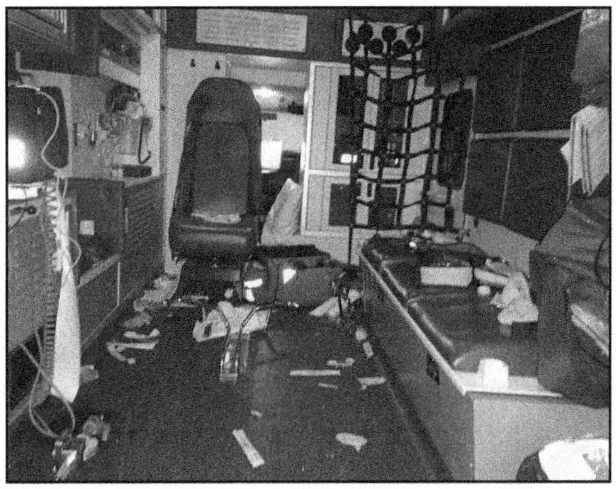

Rural EMS – making a difference in trauma care

The ideal team requires the right people and for specific calls we need the right leaders. With the right leader, we can overcome anything we face together while working, or find a solution to an unfavorable alternative. Most of our EMS calls are relatively minor, or not stressful in the grand scheme of things. However, exceptional circumstances do occur. Everyone on the team has an important role. It does not matter if one is a volunteer firefighter, an operator of the "Jaws of Life" an RCMP officer, or any one of the medical crews involved in the event (ambulance or STARS), for we all have an important role to play in changing patient outcomes.

We need to become a team despite not ever having worked together in the past. We get one chance to make things work on scene, so we must leave our egos, prejudices and negative attitudes behind. That's how we make a strong rural trauma team on any given highway or in any rural location. We become one highly functioning team and we work together for the benefit of the patients and everyone involved in the incident.

Trauma teamwork is mentally challenging and includes trying to figure out the mechanism of injury (MOI), assessing the injured, and devising extrication methods. On one challenging day, I was working with my old partner, Bailey, and she was a pure angel. Her biggest priority was simply to keep me out of trouble. That was the only thing I asked of her and it was a rather big request. We had worked many calls together and no matter what we faced, I would never stop smiling when we were together.

Our job is easy most days, but the odd day we work very hard mentally, and sometimes physically, as well. On any given day, we can have emotional highs and lows, however. On every call we always talk back and forth, ensuring we are moving forward with the best treatment options. It's 110% a team effort, with mutual respect going in all directions. Each one of us has our patients' best interest in mind on every call.

On this day, we were called to a single vehicle rollover (SVR). Thankfully, there was only one person involved. Even with one patient, though, we can be pushed to our limits, and this one call made us earn our pay. We paid for it with our patient's blood, our sweat and a few silent tears after the call.

We all work off of either international trauma life support (ITLS) or advanced trauma life support (ATLS) training, both of which are designed to streamline trauma patient care, teaching us how to respond, assess the scene, make extrication adjuncts, and how to assess and stabilize patients. Our training teaches us when we should stay on scene and stabilize, or if we should transport and do as much as we possibly can on the way to the hospital. Patient care continues after we arrive at the local ER or at the trauma centres. Critical care staff, the STARS crews and the provincial air ambulance staff are all well-versed in the steps to save lives.

In this chapter I want to illustrate some very good and concrete facts. If we work together and follow clear and defined steps, we will save lives when it comes to trauma care. What is the role of ATLS, you might ask yourself, if you have never have taken the courses? Simply put, it follows some very logical steps.

This is just a quick but straightforward summary of the course highlights after attending an ATLS course conducted by Dr. Broad. I've seen many other ATLS medical directors cover these topics, and the same issues keep coming up over and over again. They include:

1. **How to prevent accidents** – *We need to promote: 1) seat belt use; 2) use of bike helmets for kids; 3) the restricted use of quads for kids under sixteen years of age; and 4) drinking and driving kills more people than anyone would expect.*
2. **How to prevent bad resuscitations** – *By being organized, practicing one's skills, preparing the room and the equipment needed, and organizing and defining clear roles for each team member.*
3. **The importance of working from the "ABCDE" approach** – *Ensuring that we cover life threats in the most logical order.*
4. **Treating the greatest threat to life first** – *During patient assessment we will come across serious and non-serious injuries and we need to prioritize them as follows: 1) bad bleeding needs to be stopped; 2) a bad airway needs to be fixed; 3) ineffective breathing needs to be fixed or intervened before you go past this problem; 4) fractures, although they can be distracting, are not usually the highest priority but part of the big picture.*
5. **Definitive diagnosis is not immediately important** – *The trauma team and the surgical staff can complete any secondary*

and tertiary care decisions. The paramedic's job is to look after threats to life. Fix the ABC and LOC concerns, and then transfer the patient to the closest trauma team via the most appropriate and efficient transport system. The patient does not need a complete head-to-toe set of X-rays, as when they reach a trauma centre they undergo radiology assessment, which often consists of a FAST U/S scan and a CT scan as soon as they are stable.

6. **Time is of the essence** – *We all know the golden hour is vital to positive patient outcomes, but it often takes several hours to stabilize and transfer patients to a trauma centre. We need to think of the best place for the patient to be monitored, ideally a location with surgical and CT access, blood banks and the best trauma specialists available. In a small rural hospital, the patient is helped, and if they become unstable, it's a big hurry to transfer them out. Sometimes this is a death sentence. Often, we will divert from the scene to the closest trauma hospital via fixed or rotary wing aircraft to shorten the transport time as much as possible.*
7. **Do no harm** – *We need to call for help early and seek expert opinions in order to provide the best patient care. Taking extra courses and seeking additional learning experiences is something everyone should do. One must also have access to essential equipment and medications, and be aware of alternative treatment options.*

I have the utmost respect for Dr. Mary Stephens and Dr. Broad, neurosurgeons who ensured we learned the order in a simple logical format.

The **ABCDE** approach is simple:

- ✓ **A - Airway with C-spine protection**
- ✓ **B - Breathing and ventilation**
- ✓ **C - Circulation and hemorrhage control**

- ✓ **D - Disability: neuro status**
- ✓ **E - Exposure / environmental control**

As the different letters are completed and checked off, one can move on. You must still ensure that interventions are appropriate, and you must always be prepared to go back and reassess the patient at any time if the patient's condition changes or deteriorates. Look for trouble, expect the worse, and pray for the best outcome.

The greatest adjuncts to patient care are: oxygen, SpO2 monitors, BP monitor, and IV access. The baseline labs are Hgb, electrolytes, BUN, creatinine and serum lactate. The two most helpful X-rays that ought to be done, if required, are a chest X-ray and pelvis X-ray. A piece of new technology that is very helpful is the FAST U/S scan, which uses ultrasound technology to identify internal injuries, structures and fluid levels. Emergency physicians are well trained in the care of trauma victims, leading to a decrease in the mortality and morbidity rate of our patients over the years.

I am reminded of a call where we were put on high alert as we were dispatched; the situation sounded very serious. The BLS crew on scene called and requested our help as soon as possible. We already had STARS on route and RCMP, fire and additional units were available if needed. As soon as we received the distress message, we increased our ground speed. The highway was clear, and the roads were excellent. It was now as real of an ALS call as we would get.

The time for us to use our advanced airway skills, pharmacology knowledge, patient assessment skills and diagnostic abilities was now. Just before we arrived, we got an ETA for STARS, and as there was no close-by hospitals with available blood or surgical interventions, it was up to us, the on-scene BLS crew and our ALS unit, and the arriving STARS crew, to be the trauma team. As we pulled up, I'm sure I said a silent prayer; we were ready to rumble. We were going to make sure the "Angel of Death" lost this battle at all costs. We didn't know what had caused the accident and it didn't matter, we couldn't change the past. But we could change the future for our patient. That was my primary and job today.

On scene, we found the BLS crew working with the fire crews on extrication. I got a quick report from the BLS crew, assessed the scene, assessed the patient and, in seconds, we had a plan. They had already done all they could do by providing oxygen, and there was literally no extra room to do any treatments. Once the patients were released from the wreckage they would go straight to the unit for advanced airway procedures, IV access and fracture care, as we had one very bad orthopedic injury that could not wait for the rest of the trauma team. We performed cardiac monitoring, took vitals, and did a very rapid head-to-toe exam. One of us would maintain the airway and the others would help with everything else.

We had basic and advanced airway adjuncts, tourniquets ready, and intravenous lines primed and flushed. I prepared the necessary medications to help capture the airway when ready. I calculated the weight, did a few medication measurements and knew we were ready to do what we could for our patient. The fact that we had travelled a considerable distance, along with the time it took to extricate the patient, had eaten into the golden hour. We still had no real interventions started, other than some bleeding control and oxygen therapy. It was a good start and that was all anyone could ask for today. The BLS staff had done everything they could and had a spine board and cervical collar ready. Normally, we would apply the collar while the patient was still in the vehicle, but it would not help our airway problems. We could not even get enough access until fire pried the vehicle apart off the patient.

I made it clear that once we laid the patient down on the spine board, we would lose the airway. We had to slide him onto the spine board and straight into the unit as soon as fire had the vehicle off him. I took over the airway care as soon as he was clear, and off to the unit we went. As soon as he was in the unit, constant suction action was required to keep his airway clear while administering high-flow oxygen. The integrity of the airway was one of the worst cases I had seen in a long time. We had to manage it, or it wasn't going to get better until it was secured with an advanced airway device.

We then did a quick review of our patient. The ABCDE approach was done. An intravenous was inserted. We stabilized a nasty extremity fracture, which helped the peripheral circulation somewhat, but it wasn't the best. It would have to do for now. The monitor and vitals were stable. The decision was made to introduce an advanced airway. As soon as extra staff from STARS arrived we would go after an airway together. It was the best hope for a positive outcome.

I felt that I could do the intubation if I had to, and I was confident I would get it in. But why risk a patient's life when the real experts would be arriving in no time? The patient needed medication for pain control and sedation but only enough to keep him from yelling out in pain. My combination therapy worked perfectly. It helped to lessen the increased BP, decrease the pain, and made it so he hopefully would not remember this time.

As soon as we heard the STARS chopper, I relaxed, and my heart rate decreased. I knew that the right help was mere minutes away. As soon as they landed, they ran to our side door. I swung the door open like I was a Walmart greeter and smiled from ear to ear. I said, "We have a bad airway. We were waiting for you." That was all I needed to say to get them to join the battle. In no time they were introduced to the patient and the team and we went to work. Everyone had a role. The STARS crew happily took over and we assisted in any way possible to get the job done. We took a collaborative approach.

Within thirty minutes, we had a secured airway, another nasty fracture aligned and thankfully had better perfusion to an extremity. We even got to help close some open lacerations. They were quickly stapled shut to slow blood loss, and the patient was reassessed and deemed ready for flight. Overall, it was a good effort from three teams of health care providers who had never worked together before. I would rate the teamwork a 10/10, and that isn't bad for a scene call.

There hopefully would be no surprises during the flight. The patient was now stable and ready for transport. We quickly loaded him into the helicopter and they were off. The clouds parted, and the sky was perfectly still as the chopper took off. It was a sight I won't ever forget. The patient was off to one of the best trauma hospitals in the world. We all gave each other a high five and declared this battle a victory. Then we looked in our unit and I glanced down at my jumpsuit, and I realized that I was covered in blood, the unit was a disaster, the equipment was contaminated, and we'd hardly even noticed. It's odd that you can be oblivious to the amount of blood on the floor. We had been so focused on the task at hand that we hadn't even notice the amount of blood on the floor.

It's part of the ATLS survey when you're looking for sources of blood loss. Yes, there had been some bleeding on this call, but you get so focused on the airway, breathing and circulation problems, as well as the deadly wet check, and then you expose the patient, only to find out there is still blood coming from the lacerations, despite your dressings. After the patient was transported, we took ourselves out of service, to get back to our base and strip the unit.

Thankfully, someone brought us a much-needed sandwich and a cold drink. We had been working for hours without a break. On bad days someone can always make us feel better through their acts of kindness: a drink, some nourishment and a big hug are all you need sometimes. We missed lunch and before we knew it we hadn't stopped for six hours. You don't plan for a disaster. You either take over control of it or it will take control of you.

Looking back, I would not have done anything differently that day and, looking ahead, I would continue to ensure that I was as prepared as possible for the next event. The practice, the hands-on training and the unit checks had paid off. I have never regretted my

ITLS, ATLS, and real-life scenario training as they have all helped prepare me for unthinkable calls.

Nothing but time will tell us the outcomes of the calls we attend to, and for more than half of these, we never learn the outcome. In a perfect world, there would be a system to track all cases, talk to the responders and give feedback to the responders about events. It would be helpful to know what outcomes are in order to improve quality of care in the future. As we perfect our care, we do our best to make the world a little better, one person, or one call, at a time.

After our bad calls we have our best friends and our puppies to recharge us.

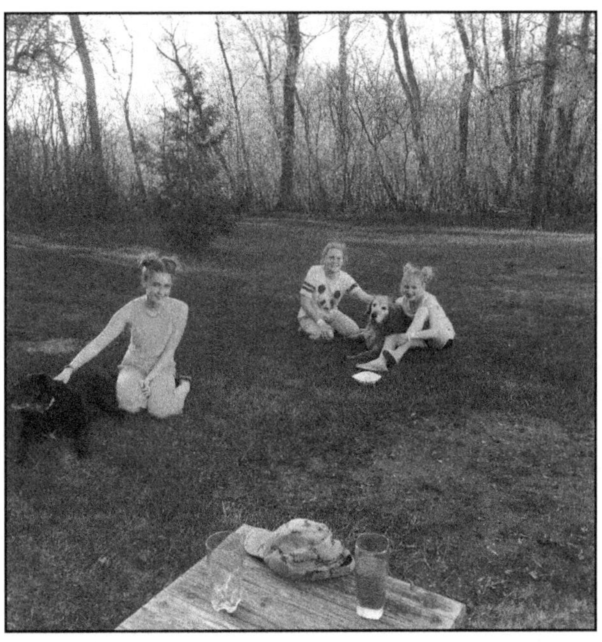

Ember and Pebbles with the kids - pet therapy is never a bad idea. Thanks Carl and Lois Franke!

Chapter 15: Teamwork Counts

"Working Together 24/7"

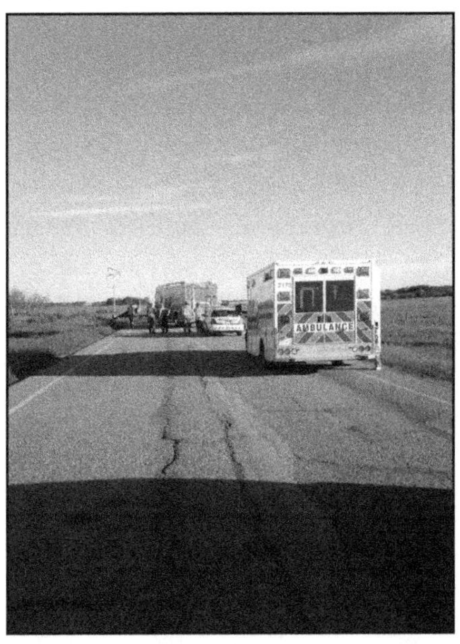

The best EMS, health care and first responder teams share one unique quality: it's the art of "teamwork." Effective teamwork is a combination of many simple skills that have been diligently practiced until they become habits. The first and greatest need for a team to excel is good communication. This is made up of interpersonal skills, body language, our tone of speech, and verbal and nonverbal communication skills.

Emotional intelligence and common knowledge play important roles in emergency medicine, especially in the stressful environment of saving lives. Within the communication system there needs to be a common language, as well as an end goal. Everyone on the team must have a purpose or a role. As in any team, they need to support each other and ensure everyone is kept safe and no one is undermined by others. It is essential that everyone knows what their individual responsibilities are, and that they know the pertinent details of the roles that every other team member play. Some roles may have overlapping or shared skills. Some people will automatically fall into a role that suits them, while others will want specific direction or a task to be delegated to them.

No matter who has which role, a harmonious and non-hierarchical attitude of all members must be in force for everyone to function together effectively. There should also be one leader for the team to function well. There are only two people who make up the responding crew on most calls. These people are assisted by backup, which can come from ground ambulances, or by air. The staff helping our team members can include: multiple volunteers, critical care teams (often composed of a surgeon, anesthesiologist, and respiratory therapist), critical care paramedics, registered nurses, as well as firefighters, and even tow-truck drivers and so on. When we respond to an incident or a call it's never just one unit or one team on scene, and there can be multiple members from many different agencies. Nothing we do revolves around the abilities of one single person. There are no single heroes, only team winners. In some cases, we lose the battle to save a life, but we always do the best we can. Some battles are lost before we start. We might fight the good fight and ends it on a swinging note. After ever bad calls, we need to look for the good in the situation, even if it's just holding a patient's hand, as we bring the family in to see them. A personal touch goes a long way.

Teams must have a leader appointed to direct procedure and process, but that leader can change as higher level of care providers arrive if it benefits the overall patient care. The leader must be chosen carefully, as their direction can make or break any team. The stronger the leader, the better the team. Poor leadership, and the team can fracture, and once things start to go south, it just spirals downward. After seeing a few bad calls that were made worse by a bad leader, you really appreciate the good leaders, and you appreciate the exceptional leaders even more. Effective leadership calls for taking control of the situation and the ability to be able to predict any number of potential adverse outcomes and make judgments accordingly, so that you can stay one or two steps ahead of potential disasters.

An effective leader must be able to take over on scene and provide guidance to all team members as they perform their respective duties. They will turn to you for help and, most of all, they need someone to be accountable for the difficult decisions that will need to be made.

Scene control begins by knowing what you're responding to ahead of time. It allows you to plan for any potential hazards that you may face, and be able to distribute resources accordingly, such as fire, rescue, hazmat, police or disaster services. When you arrive on scene, the real job of team leader starts. You need to survey the scene for potential hazards, exits and entrances. One must understand the roles of the people or resources that are already in place. Even a task as simple as parking one's vehicle must be done with consideration of everyone's safety.

On scene, we are all one team even though we are from different responding agencies. The EMS team leader is responsible for patient care. The police and fire department have other unique roles such as site safety, investigation and control of people accessing or leaving the scene. Once the EMS team leader has completed a scene assessment and a patient assessment, they must be able to produce a working diagnosis from which future decisions will be made. Then the treatment plan can be put in motion. A backup plan is always a good idea; there should always be a plan B. Make a plan, have a plan B and, some days, a plan C. The team members need to keep the leader and all other team members informed of any arising concerns or sudden complications.

As a leader you need to understand the team's expectations of the events, and you must be able to determine a plan of attack as soon as possible so they can plan they must do or what skills they must perform in order to enable a positive outcome. This lets staff plan the order of treatment. Skills are often performed under the team leader's direction.

Due to the unpredictable nature of emergency medicine, it is almost inevitable that a part or parts of a rescue can fail. The leader can make a mistake. A team member can mishear a directive and head down the wrong direction in the care being provided. A patient's condition can suddenly change. Regardless of one's role on the team, it's everyone's job to alert the leader if something is amiss and to try to correct an error before it is too late. The team needs to understand that the leader is human, and even he or she can make mistakes.

As such, a team should always offer each other support, and watch out for each other in the performance of assigned duties. Most team members are more than happy to assist others at work when they feel needed and supported. Teams are usually more productive when the members feel that they are supported by management and when the leadership offers support and provides access to required resources. It very hard to do our job and do it well if we don't have the right resources. For any team to be effective, they need to be one cohesive group. Friction among team members puts a strain on patient care. It's better just to work together and ignore the petty or small things in life. Pick your battles, but don't pick battles you can't win, unless it is to be your patient's advocate. Then it's a battle worthy of having.

Something as simple as providing nourishment, coffee and relief on a hard day goes a long way in terms of team building. I have had many bad days when someone ordered pizza or grabbed a ten from Timmy's and made our day that much more tolerable. By recognizing people's needs and by monitoring your staff, you can see who needs a break, and make sure they are cared for. A good leader knows the limitations of their staff and can judge when they need a break. They also know who they can call to support the team members when the time comes.

Team members come from all different walks of life. Some have worked for years, some are brand new, and all come with different background knowledge and skill sets. Everyone on the call is unique and will be able to offer their own expertise. There is a lot of diversity needed to deal with the different aspects of our calls, and some staff will be better at certain things than others. A good leader will recognize their team members' strengths and weaknesses. Utilizing the team for their strengths and not for their weaknesses is a sign of great leadership. A good leader knows the team. The team also knows the leader and knows what they will need and when they will need it. Members should feel free to voice their concerns so that informed decisions on overall patient care can be made.

Having fun at work is allowed. I think back to days that we worked extra hard and days that we had exceptionally difficult calls. We would always keep our cool and maintain our professionalism, but also try to make the most of the day. Expect to have some bad days, but try to look for the good things in the day, as well. Stop and smell the flowers from time to time. Take time to make others feel needed and cared for. I know for a fact that on some of my worst days the only thing that saved me was my co-workers' positive attitudes.

When we are smiling or laughing and making people smile, we are healing the broken as well. People who work high-stress positions typically make close bonds. When they enjoy each other's company, they tend to work particularly well together, and the day is more productive. Some teams find that they like to get together outside of work from time to time to socialize, and this is a great idea. Building a healthy and positive relationship with one's co-workers can make for a much more relaxed shift and it really helps reduce potential conflict. We often work four shifts with the same crew, so we get to know each other's likes and dislikes quite well.

One thing we really need to work on is supporting one another after a difficult call. The staff members who are the first to come out and greet us, to check on us after a call, are my superheroes. They are the ones who help after we return from the call to strip the unit of contaminated, bloody and dirty equipment, to help clean the kits and restock the unit. They are the ones who recharge my energy and soothe my broken soul after witnessing tragedy. They prove we are a team. During and after the cleaning, restocking, and checking of the units, talking to our co-workers about the call serves as a mental health break. Co-workers intuitively know what comes with the work we do, and the sights, sounds and residual feelings we experience after the calls are done. They are our real family.

The stressful calls and the extra time spent providing care depletes our internal resources. We need to find ways to fight the fatigue that can occur after long and stressful days. Just being on call makes it harder to sleep as well as you should or need to. It's easy to get run down after repeatedly waking up after short periods of sleep, doing emergency calls and then trying to get back to sleep afterwards. Many services still employ "first up" and "second up" crews, which means you're off-time at the station or in between calls is never really downtime or a time to relax. Urban centres have the staff and manpower to permit shift work, but while they suffer less general fatigue, it is still hard on the body. We need one or two scheduled days off to catch up on sleep and get our bodies back into a proper state.

Proper downtime makes a team more effective. We all need days off and we need to know after we leave work that we made a difference. We need supervisors who will stand up for us and managers who will support our decisions. Often, we make big decisions as a team and do it for the right reasons. I have often been called at home after a big day and been commended by my supervisor for making a difference. Such a phone call can make all the difference, given that we often worry about the calls and the decisions that we've made. It's so nice to know that we matter to others and that we have a purpose in the organization.

Spending downtime with our significant others, friends, family, and pets makes us so much more productive in the long run. The recharging of our spirit by taking in the outdoors, listening to music, engaging in hobbies and trying something new gives us the strength to go back to our next scheduled shift. But only a supportive team can make our jobs easier or worthy of the challenges we face daily, in my humble opinion. Excellent teamwork is what will make our profession soar to new heights.

The Right Partners – Teamwork Matters

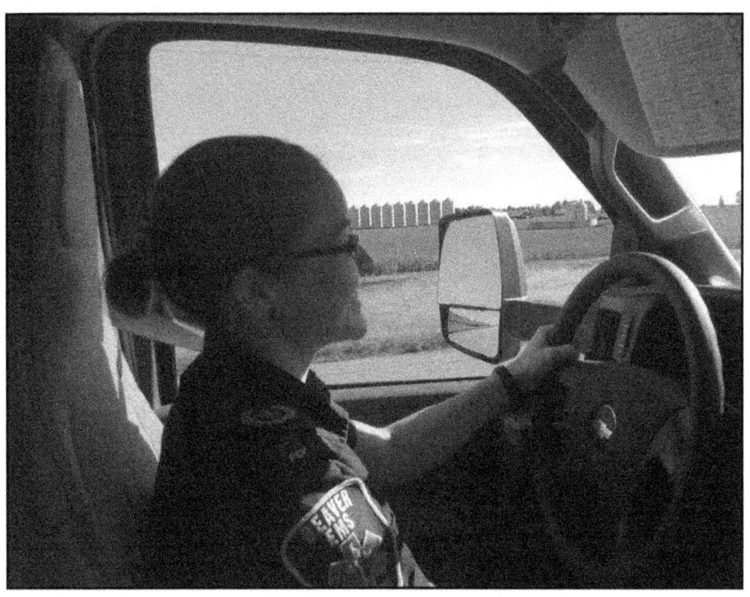

Bailey: one of the best partners I could ask for

Chapter 16: Losing Ground

"Trying to Heal a Broken Lifesaver"

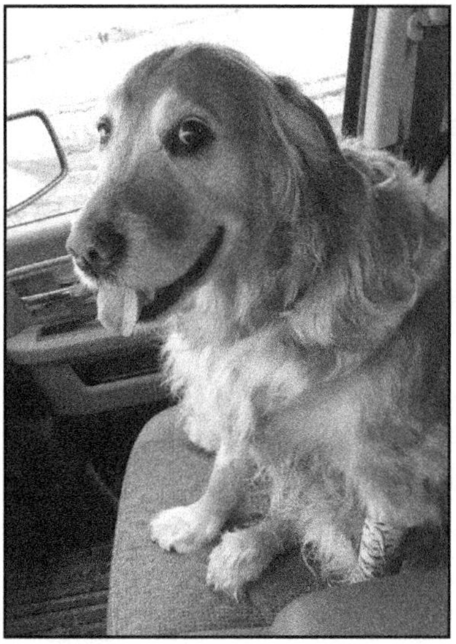

Tinsel – fighting the good fight

There comes a time in everyone's life when you need a break: a refreshment break, a nourishment break, a time-out-from-life break, or simply a brain break. At a certain point in my life, I needed to go somewhere that had no phones, no pagers, no responsibilities and no more pain. My biggest break in my life would come after a completely terrible event. I had my East Coast holiday all planned out: I was going to visit my best friend who was fighting cancer. All in all, he was doing okay post-surgery and thankfully was making the best out of such a bad situation. So often, we see our patients, our friends and our co-workers fighting terrible diseases and it takes a toll on us. That stress is cumulative somedays and other days we put it on a shelf. Some days, the shelf holding our life up simply breaks apart. Then we fall and crash when we hit the ground. Picking up the pieces is no trivial process and putting them back together is harder still.

I have often wondered why some people are prone to more misfortune than others. Why do some people seem to get knocked down more in life than they are picked up, and why do others seem to get away scot-free when they really shouldn't? I would have never predicted that the road I was heading down was going to end up hurting me more than anything I'd ever faced in my life. But fate planned my holiday to save me when I would be at the lowest point of my life. Let me just say, "No matter how hard life hits you and knocks you down, get back up, don't quit and *do not* give up."

A few hours after losing my dog Tinsel, I simply had to get on the plane and leave the world behind me. It was not one of my finest moments. I was broken, I was hurt, I was lost, I was devastated, but I managed to get back up. Losing Tinsel was like losing a child. In many ways, she was just that; she was my kid. Sadly, only a few lucky people were privileged enough to meet her. The whole world should have had that opportunity, for she was an once-in-a-lifetime gift. This is her story. Her story is one of courage, determination and love like no other. To forget her is impossible. The pain is worthy of every good memory. I will take the pain, for every tear of joy brings me closer to being a better person. It never goes away, but it will always keep me going.

No matter what we did, we could not stop the aggressive tumor that was killing Tinsel faster than we could patch her up. It was a losing battle right from the start, but we never knew what we were fighting until it was over, and she lost the battle for her life. Some battles were never meant to be won and this was one of them. At some point on that fateful day, I called my friend Troy to tell him that somehow, someway, I would make it on that plane to see him. I might not have any clothes packed, no money or anything but what I had on my back, but I was getting on that plane. Sadly, I would be flying missing one big chunk from my heart, but I had to get on that plane. It was the only thing I could do after being hurt and broken. I was too hurt to face the world.

Pebbles was not coming with me; she was going to be cared for by my friends while I was away. I had arranged it all before the terrible weekend unfolded. They would also look after my place. All I had to do was to grab my passport and board the WestJet flight heading east to the ocean of tranquility. It was not going to be a very happy trip, but it was happening the way it was meant to be, I was almost certain. Ironically, on the flight, I met a nice couple, and after a short discussion I found out that the man had just lost his dad. So, I was not the only one in pain on that plane that day. Then I found out they were not even able to sit together. I quickly fixed that problem and soon they were sitting side by side. I needed to mourn on my own, just as they needed to be together. I made a friend for life even on my worst day. I only wish I could have done more for him.

I think that sometimes we are meant to grieve away from where traumatic events happen. This trip away from my home with my good friends supporting me from afar would let me rebuild myself so that when I returned, I might be able to function in a somewhat normal fashion. Thankfully my best friends Troy, Bonnie and my retired manager, Joanne, knew what I needed. That was simply someone to cry with and someone to have my back as I tried to come back from this horrible situation. That was what I needed the most. People who made sure I was safe, when I was so vulnerable. When you're that low, you're never looking around for hazards or dangers as you would normally.

It all started one evening a few weeks previously: I had just returned from walking my golden retrievers. It was a normal walk; for a bit of time, I had lost sight of Tinsel as she was always running off and swimming, chasing sticks, or just doing whatever tickled her fancy, while Pebbles was on guard, ensuring that no predators bothered us. I thought everything was normal until I got them home safely and we went downstairs to end our day. Suddenly, Tinsel started having an atypical seizure. It was very real and scary, as I know the many causes of seizures. It was also different, as Tinsel was part of my family and not just a random patient. When its family, it's so much more real.

I had seen seizures probably a thousand times and this was very atypical in its appearance; it affected only her head and her jaw was twitching, almost like she was experiencing small electrical shocks. I laid her on my bed and waited it out, as I was sure it would soon be over. Just like that, it ended, and she needed a rest. I texted my friend, a vet in Oyen, and asked her what she thought. If she wasn't four hours away she could've helped me. I then called the on-call local vet and explained what just happened. She seemed confident that it was not something we needed to deal with tonight. We theorized that the seizure could have been caused by toxins or a tumor, but we could only guess at that point.

I wondered if Tinsel had gotten into some poison or something, as people throw garbage everywhere, and I wondered if it was possibly someone's drugs she had gotten into. Tinsel the Terminator was in trouble. I could never have imagined that this was the last month I'd have with my lady. Pebbles and I both counted on her for backup, and if you ever had the chance to see the two golden retrievers together, you knew they were a team. They were my team.

A week or so later, Tinsel had a second seizure. It was very short but still an atypical seizure. I had been worried before, as it had been an isolated occurrence, but mow I was starting to get scared. I had seen thousands of sick patients and had a list of differential diagnoses for seizures a page long. I had no idea that I was completely missing the real reason she was having the seizures. In humans, we often see seizures in patients with low blood sugar, as medication-induced reactions and reactions to medication withdrawal. I kept watching her, and treating her just as special as ever, but she was slowly changing. She became more of a loner with her head always in the corner. That was not Tinsel. She was usually at my side, watching my every move, even when she was supposed to be sleeping. Tinsel had always been my guardian angel. She had to be in pain.

Less than a week later, she had a third seizure and I knew then that something was very wrong. I carried her to the truck and drove to the vet clinic with purpose. I had to work nights in the ICU, but this was my first priority. I carried Tinsel into the clinic and had a vet at her side in seconds. They took a blood sample on arrival and her blood sugar level came back very low. It remained low on retesting, but she seemed to get better, so I took her home. I took her blood sugar before I went to work, and it was only 2.7 mmol/L. She seemed okay, and I reluctantly headed off to work and prayed she would be okay.

I put Pebbles in charge, but Tinsel also was doing her best to keep up and do her job as normal. Before I walked out the door, I took her blood sugar one more time as I didn't believe it: her blood sugar was less than 3.0 mmol/L, which was low but not critical. I was baffled. I wondered if it could be a strange endocrine or brain tumor, but I just didn't know. That night was very busy and anything that could happen did. At some point, I managed to run a stretcher over my big toe and that was the last straw. I almost cried but I just kept walking. I got the current patient settled and kept working but I was not in a good head space. I was in pain and I knew Tinsel was in trouble and I was terrified. She was hurting, too. We were both hurting, but my pain could be fixed if I could find a volunteer to rip my big toenail off. It was not going to be as easy a fix with Tinsel.

I got home from work that Friday morning and, to my relief, Pebbles and Tinsel were looking out the window, waiting for me. They always met me at the door as happy as two pups could be. They were both there, jumping up and hugging me, until we got in the truck to go for a walk and a quick vet visit. The vet assessed her, and the morning's blood sugar was 2.3 mmol/L, and I took her home and got into bed. The vet called sometime later that morning and she was concerned. She felt that something was wrong even though she wasn't sure of the cause, and she wanted to see Tinsel back at the clinic for the day, so she could run some more tests.

I reluctantly took her back and they admitted her. I also knew she was in trouble, but I still didn't know how very serious it was. I visited her again before my next twelve-hour night shift in the ICU. Tinsel was still sick but doing better; the IV dextrose was running constantly, and seemed to be helping. For some reason they still could not keep her blood sugar levels in a normal range. I had gone out and bought some beef jerky for Tinsel and for Natasha (the vet), as she would need extra energy to keep up with my little lady. Tinsel was normally so full of energy, but this day she was not ready to go home just yet. She looked to be sad and in pain.

On Saturday morning after my night shift, I went to check on her again. I took Tinsel for one more pass and then we went to Timmy's and I spoiled her again. We went on a little road trip, but her blood sugar crashed again, and I had to take her back sooner than I wanted to as she needed help. Natasha hooked her back up to the IV and I left her in the hands of a great team, even though Tinsel wanted to come home with me. I had to tell her she needed to stay, and she understood that I couldn't stay there with her.

That evening, I visited her and gave her a hug and apologized to the staff. I just had to see her again and make sure she was okay. From there, I went to ER and got them to surgically remove my angry toenail. It was a bloody mess and I'd have to say rated a 7/10 on the pain scale. Once it had been frozen and removed, the pain lessened, and the throbbing went away, and now it was just bleeding, which was not a big deal. It was a very bad night for obvious reasons. I had lots of extra blood, and I didn't think I was going to get stabbed or shot anytime soon so bleeding was sort of therapeutic. Still, I took the night off work and told them to mark it down as a mental health night or a sick night, whichever one they wanted, but I wasn't coming in to work. My co-workers understood. They all knew Tinsel, and they knew me.

On Sunday morning, as soon as we could bail her out of lockup, Pebbles and I took Tinsel home again for a short time. Her blood sugar crashed again in no time, despite the extra treats. Back to the vet's she went to get another D5W IV and surprisingly it wasn't enough, so Natasha cranked it up to D7.5W, which was something I had not seen except in newborns. Natasha and her staff were busy but took the time to spoil Tinsel as much as possible. That night, I had another bad night. I had very bad dreams, and I somehow knew the next day was going to be a day from hell, but I had no idea that hell was going to be worse than I could ever have imagined. My dreams would not stop, even in the light of the day. Even when I woke up, the nightmare was all too real. Hell was coming for us. It was too late to change course.

I woke up Monday morning, and I knew it was Tinsel's last day. I knew she was in pain and despite the vet's best efforts we were losing the battle. I just didn't know the why of it. I went to my gun locker, got out my rifle and my bullets and I told my friend it was my job or the vet's and there were now no other options. The miracle we needed was not going to happen. Somehow, heaven had simply run out of them. We had run out of any chance to fix her and heaven had no miracles left today. I just knew in my heart she was in extreme pain. I also knew she was in a terminal battle for her life and that was not something anyone could fix. I still could not believe how my life had been affected by this miracle dog. She was put on this planet for a reason. She had come into my life when I needed help and she saved me from some very bad nights. She always broke down my barriers and took away the pain. I just could not fix her despite trying my best.

First thing Monday morning, I tried to take her out of the clinic and the staff said no. I asked to speak to Natasha and she told me that Tinsel's blood sugar was critically low as she had pulled out her IV accidentally during the night. She said I couldn't take Tinsel, as it wasn't a safe or good idea, but I could not bear the thought of Tinsel dying in a cage without seeing the outside one more time. Thankfully, Natasha could see my desperation and she knew how much I loved Tinsel. I was determined; I had to take her home one last time. In the end, she was not going to win the battle for her life, but I would do anything for her to get one last shot at freedom and to feel the fresh air one last time.

I was going to ensure she got to inhale the fresh air and feel the wind on her face if it was the last thing I did. I was taking her out. Natasha understood totally. She promised to stabilize Tinsel and told me I could come pick her up at noon. I said how about one o'clock and promised I would keep her safe. I only had a few more hours with my lady and I wanted to make them count. I also had a flight to catch tonight and I was having trouble functioning from so much emotion. I still needed to pack. I didn't know how I would survive without Tinsel. It didn't seem real.

Packing was the last thing on my mind. I could not think about leaving Tinsel in distress, and I would never leave her to suffer alone. She had saved my life and I was determined to help her, but we had run out of options. Our miracle never came. If anyone deserved a miracle, it was Tinsel. She gave unconditional love to everyone her whole life and now it was going to end.

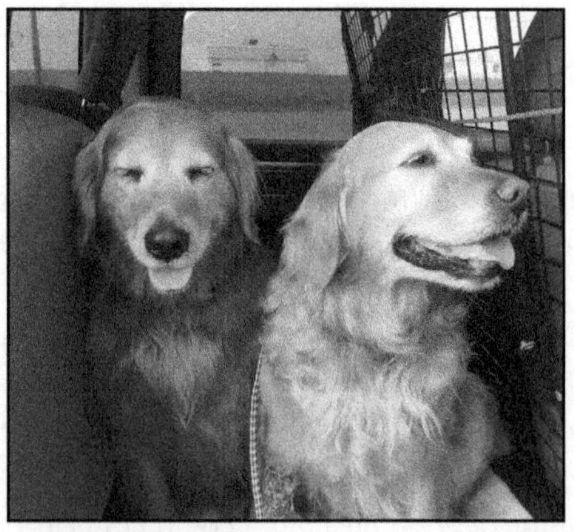

Pebbles was so happy as they got to take one last trip to Timmy's together

On Monday afternoon, I took Tinsel on one last trip with me. Louise, my close friend, and I took Pebbles and Tinsel to Timmy's. I had always bought treats for both golden retrievers when I went there, but today was special. I got Tinsel a steak panini and a grilled cheese sandwich with bacon. I knew she needed to bring up her blood sugar levels, and food was the only way I could give her more time. Afterwards, she got out of the truck west of the local Walmart, and she found the perfect stick to chew on, but she just didn't have the energy to run anymore.

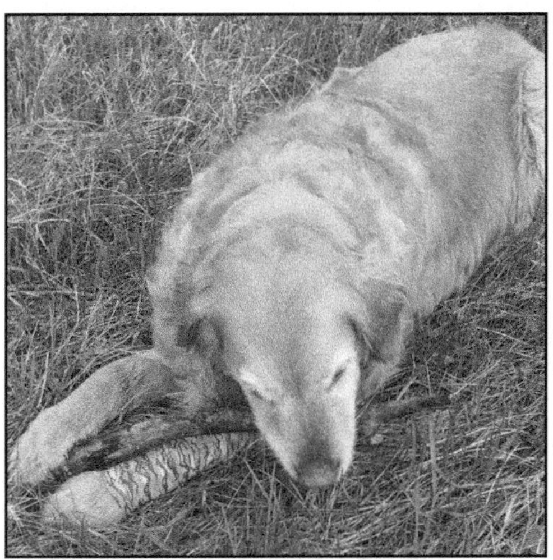

We got one last taste of freedom and it was worth it

She lay down and chewed on the stick and watched us watching her. I knew we didn't have much time. We took her home and I got one more special hug and she got to visit with the rest of her family. I lay down and she rested in my arms. Even Socks the cat gave her a hug and showed her the utmost respect. All animals know pure love. In less than twenty minutes, she was out of gas. We were in real trouble. But she needed to take one more trip. I knew it was now or never. I would move a mountain if I had to so that Tinsel would get one more chance at freedom.

This was going to be our last trip and it was going to be special. I carried Tinsel out to the truck and put her in the front passenger seat. I took off down the back roads, and I rolled her window down and let her feel the wind on her face one last time.

As soon as I got to the familiar gravel road where I liked to walk with the golden retrievers, I got her out and let her go for one last run. She ran through the ditch, into the field and back through the water. Tinsel loved that water. She held her head up high with pride and joy. We had faced many hardships together and we had beaten everything that life had thrown at us until today. I had faced a few very bad months due to my work life catching up to me, and with the help of Pebbles, Tinsel, a psychologist and my close friends, I had made it through the worst of times. I might never be the same again, but I was alive. Some days, that was as good a start as you could hope for.

As I watched her run, I had to accept that we were losing her, and nothing could stop the oncological disease from progressing, as it was too aggressive. I was losing the most incredible golden retriever I had ever met in my life. When she had her last great run, she came back to me and I lifted her back into the truck. She had gotten her wish. I quickly took her back to the vet clinic and I knew Natasha would be waiting and ready to help us. I didn't want to take her back as I knew it was the end, but I couldn't let her suffer. If I could have given my life for her, I would have, but it was not the way life worked. Somehow, I would get through this hell of leaving her behind. Somehow, I would move on. But it was not going to be easy. It was going to take time. And the real hell still awaited me; even more pain was to come.

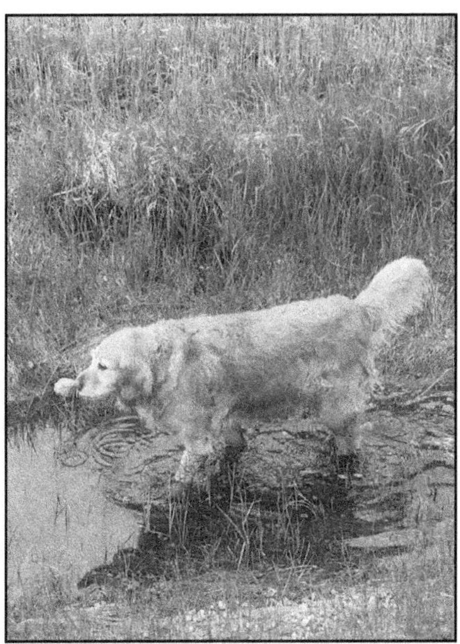

Some heroes have four legs

When we got back to the clinic, I carried Tinsel in and called for help. Natasha came to my rescue one more time as Tinsel had critically low blood sugar levels. I held her close. She wasn't physically responding anymore, but she was still looking at me. I could feel her heartbeat. I could feel her endless love. Natasha returned with an IV of glucose and dextrose and syringed it in her mouth as quickly as possible.

At the same time, Hilary was doing a surgical procedure on the table beside us with her assistants and let us do what we had to do on the clinic floor beside them. It was something I will never forget. Palliative care was our only option, but I knew she would not survive unless she was free to run and to live. We moved into a private room and I held her to my heart. She held my heart until the last second and then she let me go and I had to let her go, too. I could not let her live-in pain. We had to say goodbye. We had no options left. None at all. "Goodbye, my lady," was all I could say.

I carefully took off her collar and left her with the clinic staff. I went to my truck and Pebbles and I drove home. We both had just lost our best friend. God, I wish I could have saved her, but all I can do now is be thankful for every minute that I had her at my side.

Soon afterwards, I got a message from Natasha. It meant so much to me. It read, "I can't say it was my pleasure, but it definitely was my honour to spend time with such a star dog in her last days. She went very peacefully, and on her terms (after one last car ride). It breaks my heart that I can't fix them all, but in truth, you fixed her a long time ago by giving her freedom and love for so many years. I will not forget her. Hugs."

I replied, "I don't even know how to thank you for the weekend of hell, but you made it better, even if we lost the battle for a precious life, but we saved one very important soul. I've seen many disasters. I've worked on thousands of people, but the last weekend was the worst I've ever went through. I'm still heartbroken. I can't believe how fast she got sick. I would have done anything for her but let her suffer. She somehow came into my life and we hit it right off. We went everywhere with Pebbles. These goldens were my protectors. Tinsel sucked the worst badness out of this world. The dead kids and the repeated death and suffering we see daily at work. She helped to dissolve what evil people do to each other. She took it all away. She took it all and never even missed a heartbeat. I wonder if, perhaps, she took on too much and if it is possible that she absorbed others' poison, as the sacrifice that had to be paid. I swear she paid that price with honour and bravery like no one else I have ever seen. She was Tinsel the Terminator to the end."

Most people will never know how special she was, as they never spent time with her. I was happy that the staff at the local veterinary clinic got to meet her. Some people may be thinking, "But she was just a dog." They will never know how wrong they are. My book about her, *Between Life & Death*, (my second book) will hopefully show people that there is good in the world and that perhaps there is still hope for us all. Natasha, you were one of the good people in our lives.

Many people do not realize the miracles veterinarians such as Natasha and her staff perform helping sick and injured animals every day. When I left, I could not talk to anyone at the clinic. I walked out of that room and all I had left that mattered to me was my Pebbles. The next morning, I sent a thank-you message to Natasha and I said that I had been on a plane all night. I was crying still. My love for animals and life is as big as my heart. Again, thank you, Natasha, and please thank your co-workers for me as well. I really felt I was bugging you all, but I made a pact with Tinsel: if she saved my life, I would save hers. I didn't quite live up to my part, but I sure tried. Thank you for everything.

We all did everything we could for Tinsel, and that night Robyn helped me pack before my flight out east. My grieving would be done in the air and later by walking on the beach and looking out at the ocean. I believe it was meant to work out that way. This week away started the healing process. It was so comforting to have my friend Ray there on the plane with me. Together we went and made the best of our holiday after a very long and painful weekend.

When I was lying by the ocean when I got a message from one of my co-workers. It meant so much to me:

"Oh Dale. I am holding back tears for you. I can only imagine how much you are hurting. She was a lucky dog, who had the best life imaginable with you. She was one of the happiest, luckiest dogs I know. Keep your chin up and give Pebbles all the love she can handle today."

Over the next week, I would receive over three hundred personal messages showing love, kindness and friendship. It helped lessened much of the pain. I cried until I could not cry anymore and somehow, I made it back to a good frame of mind. My friends are my family, and for that I'm forever grateful.

Chapter 17: Helping a Friend

"Sometimes We All Just Need a Friend"

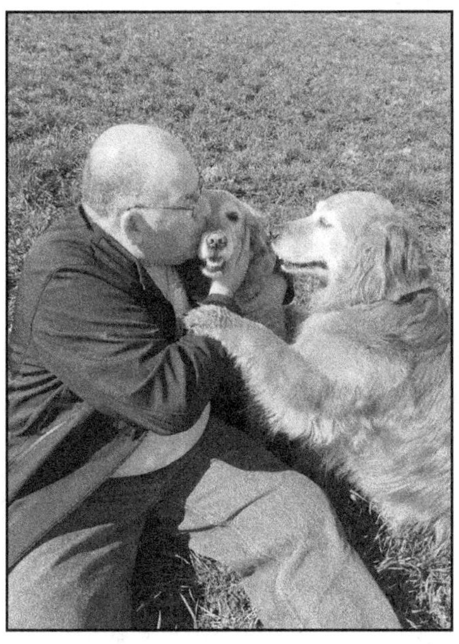

One thing we often forget, or fail to realize, is that we have friends who are willing to help us 24/7. Losing Tinsel was not easy to get over. Only time helps lessen the loss. Fortunately, I have people at my side who helped me through it. But what about the people who suffer in silence? Many of us are too proud or too scared to ask for help. It takes a lot of effort to ask for help when you are someone who constantly helps others. Several years ago, I realized we were failing our co-workers who were in distress. Even worse, I realized we had lost some of our fellow co-workers without knowing that they had succumbed to the hazards of working in EMS. By some miracle, it has finally been recognized in recent years that potential mental health risks and hazards exist associated with the profession. We must try our best to help our EMS co-workers and friends in need, before it becomes a terminal problem.

Our association and governing bodies have also realized the crisis. Help comes, but for many it's too late. My circle of friends and I are on the right road to helping each other, despite a slow start. We needed to figure out that we were at risk before we could find a way out of stressful situations without undergoing further personal injury. As an organization, we are finally able to spread the message. We mustn't waste time looking back and say that we should have done something. All we have for sure is today. We must plan today how to change tomorrow, so that those affected get a chance to see the future. Moreover, we can make the future brighter for our newest members and our current members.

It's easy to reflect on one's worst days, but it is sometimes difficult to sort out why they were so bad. The tragedies of others can be toxic. What will affect one of us, will not affect all of us the same for multiple reasons. That's when our friends show their true colours, and show they care for us just as much as they care for themselves. Sometimes we care for our partners more then we care for ourselves, truth be known. The truth is that we are often too busy looking after our patients and our partners to recognize that we may also be injured mentally, physically, emotionally or spiritually. On the bad days, we scrape through on nothing short of a miracle or by divine intervention. We make it through some very bad events throughout our careers. I would have to say that we've likely all been saved by our "guardian angel" from time to time.

I thought about it some more and realized three of my past co-workers were diagnosed with post-traumatic stress disorder (PTSD) and also showed the effects of compassion fatigue. We now know what we used to refer as "burnout" was actually PTSD. No one even knew it existed at the time. I've only needed to use my lifeline twice, but times it was for a very good reason. I also realized that I can honestly look back and say I have had a few times in my life when I needed help more than anyone else in my life. After some bad calls and some bad days, I needed some help myself. When the effects of PTSD start calling the inside of your brain home, it's not a great feeling.

My PTSD was like an uninvited guest who visited more often than I wanted them to, especially when I really needed to sleep. After missing too much sleep, the effects just compound themselves. You begin to have trouble managing your day-to-day life, and nights become your mortal enemy. There is no shame in admitting that you need help. We have more friends than we realize! I called a friend and in no time, I had help and somebody at my side. This world can be hard on many people for many reasons, and it's okay to not be able to take it anymore. But before you realize that you need help, you may feel utter helplessness, and it can be overwhelming. The first step is recognizing the pain in the mirror and feeling the helplessness in your soul.

As of this writing, tragically, about fifty-seven EMS workers have taken their own lives. They never told anyone. They never asked for help or their cries for help went unanswered. That number doesn't include rescuers we don't know about or the ones who quit EMS after a bad call and never got the help they needed. It also does not include those who drink alcohol in excess or abuse prescription medications to take away the pain. No amount of medication or liquid courage can dull this sort of pain that burns away at our inner spirit. Then one day it hit me: I was almost one of those numbers, and I didn't even know it. When one is troubled mentally, physically, emotionally or spiritually, one loses the ability to sense danger. I challenge anyone who reads this to take the time to stop and call a friend who seems "off" lately and lend them your ear if they need to talk. Provide them with the time to talk openly and honestly, and then chances are that you'll both be able to sleep better tonight.

We need to make sure our EMS family members feel supported when it matters the most. Start a conversation after the hard calls, or during the cleanup of your unit. Please take the time to greet your co-workers when they come back to the base. Give them a time out, if needed, and help them clean, restock, and recharge. After tragic calls, follow up with them a few times in the weeks and months that follow. Text them and make sure they know that they matter to you. Let them know that they have someone to talk to who won't judge them. The act of sharing is a huge step. Sharing the pain, the guilt, the pressure to be 100% on top of things, when you feel so down. Know you all have someone on your side who will help pick you back up.

We need to practice self-awareness and self-assessment when we are not feeling ourselves. If someone is reaching out to help you, let them help. Thank God for speed dial and an address book with a list of friends in it. But don't abuse your friends by asking for their advice and then not taking it. You owe them that much if they bothered to help you. Don't make them suffer, as well, by making them think that they never got through to you. That would not be fair. That is one of the worst things you could do to a friend. If you need help, take it, knowing it comes from the heart.

The role of an EMS worker has traditionally been to help others in need, but we have not been good at looking after ourselves. We have not been good at looking for the signs and symptoms of compassion fatigue in responders dealing with pain, hurt, and suffering. If we have some good days in the middle of a bad stretch, we will heal ourselves. Working with the right partner and with the right team, we can also watch out for each other. We can share the pain and give each other breaks from life's troubles. We have realized that we, as first responders, are not immune to the effects of PTSD, even if we think we are. It only takes one call to affect us. When that happens, we become a victim as well.

The greatest gift to me was when I knew Sarah was back as my EMS partner. We would have Salt or Pepper working with us, so it would be a blast. I spent two months as Sarah's mentor and then I was going on permanent vacation. On her first shift, I passed her my drug pouch and said, "You're the boss, I'm the backup." She smiled and nodded. I had no doubts about her ability; she'd had the confidence to make the shift to ALS a long time ago. All she needed was the experience to make the transition—experience based on the real world and not protocol or training scenarios.

A true mentorship exists to help someone who is still learning figure out their role in an organization, to guide them as they sort out what their own strengths and weaknesses are. Everyone needs to find their groove. Some practitioners are aggressive, some passive. There is room for both, in my experience. Some days you need to be the boss and others you are okay to just sit back and watch the world go by. Pick your battles, but pick battles you know you can win. Even better, pick battles that are worth dying over. I have a few solid rules and the most important one is to protect my partner at all costs.

After our unit check, we headed to Timmy's, and on the way, I did a bad thing: I stopped to hug my puppies. They needed me, and I needed them. I also wanted Sarah to meet my new miracle; her name was Ember. She was not a golden retriever on the outside, but she was 110% golden on the inside. That's what matters the most. We gave them an extra treat and off we went.

I enjoyed working with Sarah. During this shift we both needed some coffee, and today we had Pepper as our partner. It was so refreshing to sit back, and share our stories of our personal and work adventures. We didn't have the time or the energy to be negative. I was thinking as we drove into the Timmy's parking lot that Pepper didn't understand how close my bond was with Sarah, but she would soon.

Our first call was a fall at a local seniors' lodge. Those are the good calls as the old folks just love to see us, and they are always so grateful. On arrival, we were greeted with a quick history as we walked toward the patient's room with our stretcher and our kits. Sarah and Pepper were in the lead with me following behind. As we enter the patient's room, we saw trouble. We saw a frail-looking lady, who appeared to weigh about thirty-five kilograms if that. The history was rapid weight loss and malignant cancer. We looked at each other and knew that the patient's outcome was grim, at best. She smiled at Sarah and said, "I just need a little boost, dear." We all smiled back, and Pepper replied, "That's our job." We are more than happy to give the good people a boost.

We assessed the patient and, as carefully as possible, helped her back into her recliner. She was adamant that she didn't want to go to the hospital and that she just needed help to get off the ground. Cancer can be such an unforgiving and unkind disease, but still our patient could smile and be thankful to us. We completed our examination and checked her vital signs and I said to Sarah and Pepper, "I'll be right back," and went to talk to the director of the home. I knew she would know the patient's story, and she would give us her words of wisdom as well.

The short of it is that the patient most likely had a pathological fracture of her hip and she knew that she wouldn't leave the hospital once she got there, for it would be a one-way trip. I told the director our concerns and advised her of the patient's wishes. She wanted to spend a little more time at home, and it was easy to see how much that meant to her. Her room was so organized and cozy. When you walked into it, you immediately felt the warmth. We made a backup plan. We couldn't force her to go, as she wanted to stay where she was, and she refused pain control and transport, and we respected her wish. We knew it wouldn't be long until she fell again, or otherwise lost her mobility, and we would get called back. Even if it was one more day, it was important to her to stay, and, thus, an easy decision for us, even when we knew she had to be in pain.

We asked her to sign a cancellation form, and ensured that the home care staff, director and family were all happy with the decision. A home care team was making patient rounds in the building that day, and they promised to keep an eye on her. They, too, knew that it was just a matter of time. She was seated in the perfect position so that she could watch the birds outside her window. As we walked out, she was simply watching and waiting for the birds to come back after all the commotion faded away.

The little birds would give her peace for the next few hours, which to someone with not much time left, was invaluable. I thought back too many years ago when a patient asked me for one small favour. I said, "What can I do for you?" Sadly, I just don't know if he got it. All he wanted was one more day. I prayed that night that he got his wish, but I never found out if he did. As we walked out of the nursing home that day, we all shed some tears. It was one of those moments we don't plan for but are thankful for when they come along.

The rest of the day was so much fun. Every time we got another call, someone quickly acknowledged it and we were off. One person did the ePCR, while the other drove and planned the call. It was so positive to have everyone working together to have a good day and no matter the next call, we greeted it with a positive attitude. We all gave each other the encouragement to do the best we could, no matter the case or the difficulty of the call. Some days, I didn't want the shift to end, as the work was therapeutic. At work, we have friendships, but once we get home we often just have silence, and on bad days that makes for a long night. Some days, just having a partner, even if you're busy working, gives you piece of mind knowing that you're safe and you have someone to watch over you. That's a true partner, but also an EMS friend for life.

Our last call was complex, but a rewarding call. It was an ALS transfer of a septic patient. We walked into the local ER and they immediately requested help. In no time, we were mixing medications, preparing an advanced airway, and ensuring that the IVs were okay before we initiated transport. When you're providing multiple IV boluses to a very sick patient, it's easy for your IVs to fail. Throughout the call, I tried my best to stay back and observe, then realized it would be more beneficial for me to do the work and let Sarah be the boss, as that was what she needed the most practice with. Learning to be a mentor is harder than you'd think.

After we initiated the transport, the patient's vital signs were trending up favorably. When you see the urine start to flow into the urinometer, it is a good sign. In critical care, we need to measure the volume of urine produced by the kidneys and it's measured more frequently in sicker patients. We can gauge how well our resuscitation is going by seeing the kidneys working or not. You always smile when you see the urine is yellow and clear, knowing the renal system is getting the blood flow it needs to keep the patient's body system working. With the miracle of life-saving antibiotics already initiated, all we had left to do was to titrate vasopressors to keep the patient's blood pressure in the proper range.

It's amazing to think how much we have learned to help save septic patients from dying in the last ten years. Sarah's and Pepper's careers will hopefully see many more advances in patient care. With medicine, we constantly see changes, and the only way to keep up with the changes is to maintain a positive attitude, and to keep learning. To know that our career demands lifelong learning, and to embrace the professional changes that will ultimately help save our patients lives.

On the way home, we had a great discussion about the last couple of days. The one thing we all agreed on was that it had been a great tour. But the moment we got back to the base, we were called back to the seniors' home. It was called in as a respiratory or cardiac arrest. As we got closer, we realized that it was the same little old lady from a few days earlier. We grabbed our LP-15 monitor and our ALS kits and made our way into her room. We were met by the staff and they helped us to her room, where we found our nice lady from a few days ago looking to be sleeping in her recliner. She looked so peaceful. She had no pulse and she was not breathing. It was exactly what she had wished for; she got her final wish. Nobody could take that from her.

We were aware of her code status, and we knew this was as far as we needed to go. Suddenly we all turned and saw the prettiest white dove at the bird feeder. It silently acknowledged us, and then it lifted off and glided away. I was raised on watching some good TV shows and the ones that came to mind right then were *Highway to Heaven* and *Touched by an Angel.* It was clearly one of those special moments. She got her final wish and was able to make peace with the world; the miracle of the birds did the rest. We made a few phone calls, and the family and staff took over. We went back to the unit and finished our electronic paperwork. Our role that day was complete. We made our way back to the base. No one said anything. It was the perfect time not to say anything.

After we cleaned our unit and counted and signed the medications over to the next crew, we met in the parking lot. The three of us sat for a spell and watched the world go by. We knew we made a difference. We had not done anything monumental or heroic that tour, but we had touched the lives and hearts of the people we helped. That's sometimes the part that people miss. At the end of the day, we are all but one family. I'd gotten some sleep last night so today I could stay awake and do odd jobs that needed to be done around home. My time was mostly taken up with spoiling Pebbles and Ember. We also had a nap on the king-sized bed with my two cats. Thankfully, they were kind enough to leave me a spot.

Days later, on my first day off in a while, I made a point to phone Sarah before I went to bed. I just needed to talk to someone. I had to know she was okay, and I really just needed to hear her voice. I couldn't explain the feeling, but it was a priority. When she answered, I knew she was okay, and I could relax some. I asked her how her day off was without us bugging her. I told how our day went. We started talking and before I knew it, two hours had passed. We talked about so many things.

We shared the good and the bad stories from the recent months. The difficult memories had slowly faded out of my conscious, though, before the call even ended. In this world of EMS, we are lucky if we can find a few soul mates with whom we can openly share some of our most intimate fears. We all need a way to express our feelings, because if we hold them in, we are only doing inner damage to ourselves. It lowers our blood pressure and relaxes our hearts when we can get rid of the excess baggage of the past days.

Before hanging up, Sarah made me laugh, telling me she was counting the sleeps until we would be partners again, and there were only three more days or 82 hours. That was as close to a perfect Christmas present I could ever have asked for, even if it was not even close to the Christmas season. I let her go on the promise that I'd call her whenever I needed to talk. That was an easy deal. I had her on my speed dial, so she was only one finger away, 24/7. As she hung up, I realized that there were more angels in this world than we ever imagined. We need to look harder for the good people and the good things in life to recharge our spirit. It reminded me of an old, wise saying, "The closer you are to the good, the further you are from the bad." That was where I needed to stay.

A lighthouse gives us peace and protection from the world.

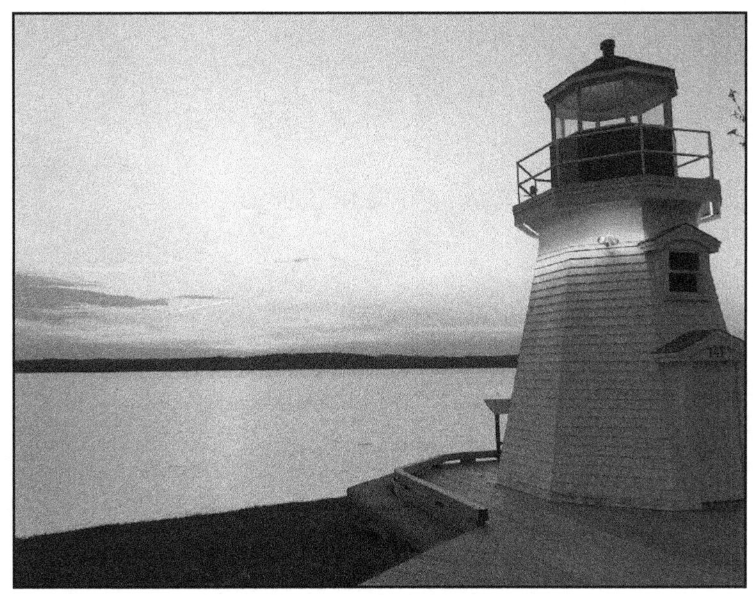

On some days, all we need is the goodness of the world to be our light!

Chapter 18: Making the System Better

"Transforming Our EMS Culture"

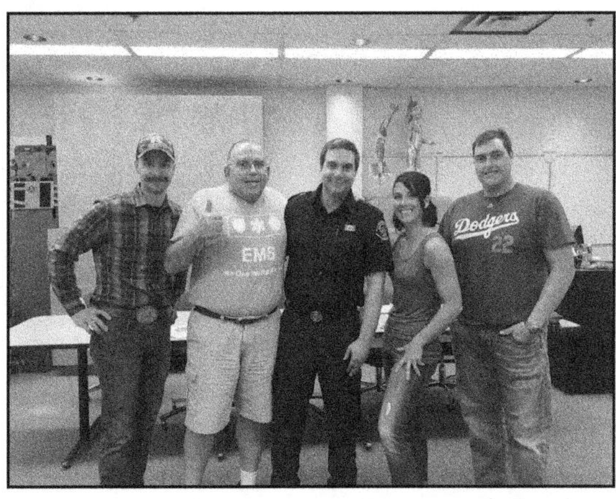

The only way to make our emergency medical system better is for us to evolve into a solid and reliable body of professionals. We need to accept changes and grow from within to become a stronger profession. We need to work as a team, no matter our rank, our training, or years of experience. We need to strengthen our education system to allow for more comprehensive learning of enhanced therapeutics and treatment modalities, and to teach our students to become the mentors of the future. We also need to increase the practical components of the education system to help our profession expand our scope of practice and not restrict our practice due to individual weaknesses. Let's collectively find the weaknesses of our profession and make them our strengths.

By working within the community, by adding specialty teams and by collaborating with other health agencies, we can provide an increased EMS presence in our communities. By also increasing our awareness of the multiple needs or required aspects of patient care, and by increasing our simulation technology and utilizing our education resources, along with our skills, we can achieve the full potential of the role that EMS plays in the health care industry. We need to include community needs in our planning and education, and we must try to meet the needs of the people we serve as best as we possibly can.

We need to examine the negative stereotype of our profession as one with a short-lived career expectancy. Anyone who has worked in EMS has seen their share of negativity, but in truth, the industry is full of positive and dedicated people who work hard to be the best EMS providers they can be. By working at forming a stronger, more positive team, we can strengthen our endurance by not wasting time with negative energy. Life is too short to waste on trivial efforts. Let's take the time needed to regroup and refocus our profession as we all enter a new era under the Health Professions Act (HPA). The HPA permits us to provide care under our own license and be accountable to our own registry body. Let's make a positive collective effort in enhancing our profession.

The new system is allowing us to be community paramedics. That's a huge step in expanding our profession. To be able to enter a patient's home and treat the patient and interact with family members is something that we have missed out on in the past. Traditionally, we were only called if someone needed to go to a hospital. Our primary goal was to transport patients to hospital for further care. Now we know there are cases were transporting the patient is not truly benefiting the patient or relieving the strain on our already taxed health care services.

If possible, we can provide the essential resources, supplementary medications and support that patients and their families need without having to go to the hospital. In the old system, we simply transported the patient, provided symptom-relief medications when needed, and then were often stuck in a busy hallway with the patient on an uncomfortable bed for hours. There are times when we have no choice but to transport, but if the patient meets established criteria for staying in their home, and the community resources and additional support are in place, we can provide the care they need in a safe and familiar environment, thereby granting patients the dignity of staying at home.

I remember a day that started out cold and miserable. There was a strong wind and driving rain, which was not common for this time of year. I was driving the PRU and Sarah was my partner. We had been to a few local schools that day, teaching CPR. I had added an extra presentation on current real-world issues, such as the Fentanyl crisis, bullying and the effects of drugs and alcohol on driving. All of these topics were among the common ways kids get hurt and killed. I figure the more education, the better when it comes to our young people.

My messages to them were simple: "Don't do drugs" and "always wear your helmet." I added: "Don't ride with drunk or impaired drivers" and "call you parents if you need to." I especially emphasized to the kids the need to be careful on quads and all forms of all-terrain vehicles (ATVs); any quad over 350 cc is so heavy that when it rolls onto someone, it can kill them. Every pediatrician I have ever met has classified quads and trampolines as deadly pastimes. All you need to do is lose control one time and you can become a statistic.

Before you ride or drive with anyone, always ensure you're going to arrive alive, or don't go. Call someone who loves you to come pick you up, if you need to. In every class lecture, we encouraged kids to participate in the discussion. I've found that if you treat students with respect and honesty, you get so much more participation in our courses. At the end of one of the courses, a few interested students came up and we arranged a tour of the base. I looked at all the students and I knew we had gotten our message across that day.

After we left the school, we headed back to the base. We were almost back when the "Tango Three" unit called for assistance. They were supposed to be on a routine transfer, and it was rather odd for us to help with simple transfers. We got the t address and acknowledged the call to our dispatchers. On arrival, we booked "Arrived on Scene" on our CAD system. We were not sure what they could be needing, so we just went in with our radios and a good attitude. With the right attitude, any feat or difficulty can be overcome.

We met Connor and Julie in the living room. A temporary hospital bed had been set up in the spare room for the patient. Home Care had been involved with the patient for a while. They had been called to transfer the patient from his home to the palliative suite at the local hospital. The patient's wishes were to go to the local hospital for the remainder of his life.

The patient was suffering from cancer and had arrived at the point where he needed to be moved to the palliative room at the local hospital. The patient had chemotherapy just over a week ago along with radiation therapy to slow down the cancer's aggressive nature. Since then, he had been vomiting and was grossly dehydrated. Connor and Julie wanted help to relieve some of the pain and maybe rehydrate him some and try to stop the vomiting. For that, we have just the right drugs. We have the time, compassion and the right people who can help. The plan was that once he was feeling a little better, we could accommodate the transfer. It would take a little time, some IV therapy skills and just the right medications. Our new role was to make the patient's day as good as it possibly could be.

Some patients want to stay at home for as long as possible, and occasionally we have patients who want their life to end in their own home, on their terms. It's a personal and family decision. There is no perfect or "right way" to pass away, but if someone can comfortably pass with proper pain control, medical support and a little extra care, it makes some people's final days on this earth a little more comfortable. Sometimes we forget, but we are all going to die one day. It's the ability to die with as much dignity as possible that is so important to many of us.

After seeing so many people at their worst, we come to understand the importance of always going the extra mile when we see the need. We quickly made a game plan and got to work. The newest anti-emetic on the market, Zofran (also known as Ondansetron), is amazing for stubborn cases of vomiting or emesis. Pain control is sometimes harder, especially when palliative patients are already on stronger medications than those we currently carry.

We often add sedatives to narcotics to make the medications more effective. A good history and a careful review of the patient's medication history will tell you what will probably work and what won't. In palliative patient care, we often need to be more liberal with our narcotic dosages, as the patients are often on high doses of pain medication already. Sadly, on this day this could compound the problem. We were privileged to be able to call the OLMC to seek their opinion on what medications or dosages to give.

In just under an hour, the patient was feeling much better and was ready for transport. On the way to the hospital, he wanted to take one more ride past the nearby lake to see the birds, feel the wind on his face and appreciate the outdoors. That was an easy request for someone who would never see the outside again. We cleared it through dispatch and we were off on a little adventure. It was something that you normally don't have the time or the resources to do, but today, we made it happen. To see someone, smile, close their eyes, take in the sounds and appreciate the smells and other wonders of the world makes you aware of the fact that so many people never get this chance. We all know and have seen patients who never got the extra time to appreciate the good things in life. Today would not be one of those days. Today we would make this patient's day memorable, despite his pain and suffering.

If only we had the resources, the people and the time, to make this happen for everyone. With the addition of the "community paramedic" role, we were on the way to making that possible. The days of "scoop and run" were gone, as was the golden rule from years past. The art of "community medicine" could now accompany ALS as a field of practice in EMS.

The key to making our EMS system more effective at the individual level is having great leadership. You can't just be a follower if you truly want to make a difference in patients' lives. Effective leadership at the management level, both during and after calls, helps to make the system more productive. That needs to be enhanced with our work ethics and patient care dedication. The more effort you put into a job, the better the result will be. If you start a job with a great attitude, your outcomes will be better than if you're harbouring a negative attitude.

If you only care a bit and only help a bit, the patient will think we don't care at all. It is essential that our patients' needs be at the forefront of our profession. We need to adhere to system rules, the patient care guidelines and keep everyone safe, all while knowing at the end of the day that we are doing the right procedure or skill for the right reasons. We need to cultivate accountability, respect for, and loyalty to the communities we serve. We need to be the people who are trusted with others' lives to do the right thing when it counts. We need to earn that respect and need to maintain it at all times.

We need to learn to appreciate both the differences and the similarities of the people in our caring profession. Many staff offer a signature personal touch to their services, and that makes us all look good in the eyes of the public. We must go the extra mile for our patients and continue to be a voice for people in need. How we approach a problem is something we might not have appreciated, as we all have different perspectives. Life itself teaches us to come at problems from different angles and look for better solutions, but we are often slow to adapt or reluctant to change our practices. It's so important to keep an open mind and to adopt new techniques to master our role in the profession.

With the nature of our industry and the desire to be the best we can be, it's important to remain humble. You will encounter people with diverse skills and knowledge to impart and you need to be open to accepting changes to your own practice. You need to be willing to let others mentor you at times and, even if you don't agree with them, you can still humbly let them speak their mind. You don't have to agree with everyone. In fact, it's okay to disagree when it comes to personal and ethical issues that we need to be accountable for. Over the years, we have seen drastic changes to our profession that have truly created a more rounded practice. Over the years, I have met many intelligent practitioners and have often learned that they had other professional education, as well. It's not uncommon to meet foreign physicians, nurses, respiratory therapists and pastors working in our field. It makes for a much more well-rounded team of professionals.

It is important that we give back to our profession. It is a selfless act to want to enhance the lives of our co-workers, students and others around us. We have mastered the art of helping others in times of distress. But ask yourself after your shift: What did you really accomplish? Can we help others in ways not already done or seen? Can we change the destiny of the next generation? There are many ways to give back to a profession, but to volunteer to mentor others is the easiest and most effective way to make a difference. All it takes is a little effort from each of us and the rewards to our profession are increased exponentially.

The most rewarding feeling or sensation is knowing you helped someone else have a better day. Simply doing extra tasks, showing you care and making sure your co-workers are okay, is all you need to do make their world a little better. After a bad call or a long day, we can do the extra things like grab them a coffee, help them with cleanup, do their paperwork for them or top up base duties. Nothing says thank you or shows people they are supported like the act of pitching in and helping them out. The world can have a negative effect on us all, if you let it. By doing the easy, little things, we can help our co-workers have a much better day.

Building on the positive skills of our co-workers and learning to appreciate the excellence they offer to their patients is so very important in our field of work. We all have our breaking points and we all need a boost from people around us. Often, when you least expect it, stress can show up, take over, and make your life that much more difficult. Our job is very demanding, both physically and emotionally, and the mental stress that results is cumulative. We need to go the extra mile for our co-workers to let them know that they are not alone. PTSD and compassion fatigue can be deadly if we let them take hold of our lives. Do whatever you can to ensure your partner is safe, and they will do the same for you on your worst day, or during your terrible long and scary nights.

After taking our palliative patient on one last joyride, I went home and hugged my puppies in the driveway. God knows I missed Tinsel, but Pebbles and Ember had mastered the therapeutic touch I needed. That evening, I thought long and hard about life and death. I missed my friends and my parents more after this shift than usual. I texted Sarah and got a text from her right away to pray for her as she was on a bad call at the time. She had gone in for an extra shift. I wished I could have been with her. That's the world we live in. It's high stress and high stakes. It's "life and death" decisions on a second's notice. I couldn't sleep until I got another text from Sarah letting me know that she was safe and well. That was the news I needed to shut off and recharge in time to face a new day, in a few more hours.

When we stand up for each other we become stronger as a team. We all need to know we are never alone.

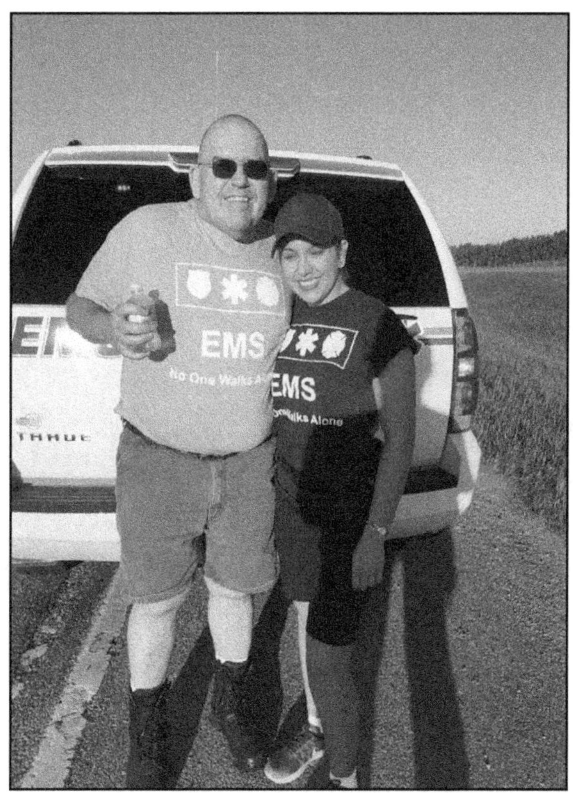

#NoBodyWalksAlone2018: We had up to 22 people walking at one time!

Chapter 19: Excellence Matters

"The Importance of Caring"

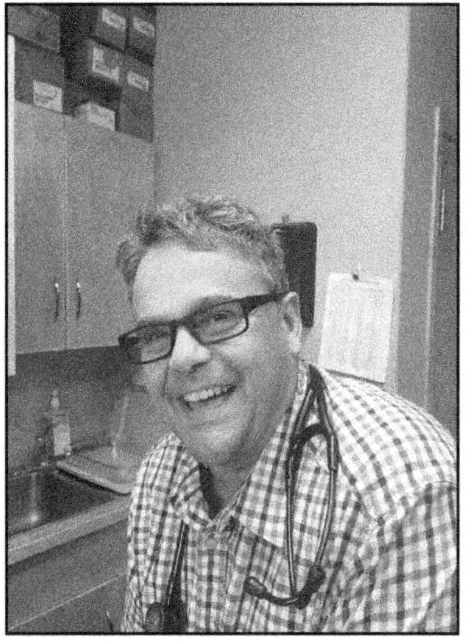

Dr. Christoff de Wit – a true friend

The only way to truly make a difference is to give it everything you have in your effort to change the world, 24/7. You might not always succeed, but your effort will not go unnoticed. It's this constant effort that is needed to change the destiny of others. It is the only real way we can affect the change needed to make the world a better place. If people just walked around obstacles, ignored people in need, and put no effort into others, it would make for a very lonely world.

As a human race, we were not created to just sit and watch time pass by, without putting in the effort to survive and to do well. In emergency medicine, we need to get our newest members to take the lead, to make changes as we constantly progress within our profession. When I look back on what I believe really makes a difference in the profession, the top things I think of are: dedication, commitment, putting in the time in order to excel, and seeking extra learning opportunities. Not every student has the ability to excel, but if you give them all the chance, they will do their best and that's a good start in my eyes. If we mentor them, they can only get better, and with time, they will master their chosen profession.

Dedication to excellence is a leading trait when it comes to learning and it is seen in many forms, including personal presentation, professionalism, and a willingness to learn. You can always pick out the students who participate in class and ask questions to clarify their knowledge, not to make themselves look smarter than the other students.

Commitment to doing whatever it takes shows the dedication needed to excel in such a demanding profession. Students who are dedicated to excellence tackle the difficult courses head-on and they seek help when they need it. They also take the role of a mentor with weaker students and you can see them helping their classmates whenever they can.

Putting in the extra time to study, to practice one's skills, to work with the other students in the class, also shows the teamwork needed to be part of a team. It was amazing to me how many days after classes, the keen students would meet and work on assignments together. They were always going above and beyond what was asked of them to ensure they were going to be successful. It was awesome to see them grasp the more difficult skills or knowledge after working hard. The one part of the course that commonly presented a challenge was EKG (ECG) interpretation. An electrocardiogram (EKG) is a test we do by applying our Physio LP-15 monitor on the patient, which then records electrical activity from the heart and produces an EKG strip that we can print off or transmit to a cardiologist for advanced interpretation. It may look easy to figure out, but it's one of the harder skills a primary care paramedic (PCP) must master.

Seeking extra learning opportunities shows true initiative. We have a set curriculum we need to teach in the classes, but it only consists of the essentials for the student to get by in the real world. For students to realize this and then choose to continue their learning shows that they appreciate the complex and dynamic nature of the profession they are entering. The simple truth of our profession is "the more you learn, the more you don't know anything," for as we learn, we realize the health care world is forever changing. The more you learn, the more you need to learn. The cycle is never-ending. As the profession progresses, we will someday have our own experts within the EMS world.

When you see the students, you taught become your co-workers, it's the biggest reward. For me, mentoring them into the EMS world was so much fun, even if it is harder than you think to keep up with the keener employees. I remember my last shift as mentor for two of the top achievers from the PCP program, Salt and Pepper. We had planned a movie night after our last shift was over. It was a good idea, even if it never happened. When we got the page for the maternity transfer, Salt and Pepper cheered, and I moaned. They both wanted to deliver a baby, and the last thing I wanted to do was deliver a baby in the back of our unit.

I had done many deliveries over my career. Most were uneventful, but I had also had some bad ones. A few times, the newborn had come out in severe distress and several went into cardiac arrest. If the baby comes out not breathing, with no heartbeat, the call becomes a big nightmare. The smallest newborn I ever delivered weighed under a pound, at less than twenty-three weeks' gestation. The infant was so small, I could hold the whole baby in the palm of my hand. Thankfully, that one made it, but many others who were older and bigger did not fare so well.

The transfer was for a thirty-eight-week gestation delivery with failure to progress, despite twenty-four hours of labour. They didn't have a surgeon on call tonight, so they elected to transfer to the closest hospital with an OR and surgical team available. The ladies wanted the call and I was more than willing to drive. My plan was to drive as fast and as safely as possible. When we picked up the patient, she was smiling during the contraction-free time. The contractions were irregular and variable in their discomfort. She would have one strong contraction and one weak one. It made me hopeful that we would not have to deliver on this call, so I was a little relieved. We loaded the patient and headed to the hospital, with our happy crew and our soon-to-be mommy on board.

We had a one-hour transport time and I would make it in fifty minutes, if at all possible. We had been driving for about twenty minutes when then the noises got louder and louder in the back, as if the contractions were getting worse. I briefly wondered if one of the two troublemakers in the back had caused this, but I knew they wouldn't have, even if they wanted to perform a delivery. As the contractions got stronger and closer together, I knew we were going to run out of transport time, no matter how fast I drove. I called back and in a matter of seconds I had Salt at my side. I said, "What are doing back there? Are you trying to make her have her baby on route? Did you start an infusion to stimulate her contractions when I wasn't looking?" She smiled and said, "We *are* having a baby, so you might as well pull over." I slowed down and found a safe place to park. I also radioed dispatch and told them our situation. They immediately dispatched a second unit, just in case we needed extra help. As I stopped, I prayed that this delivery would be as natural and uneventful as possible.

I jumped into the side door of the unit to find my co-workers already had the baby bundle open, suction ready, and heaters turned up—everyone was ready but me. I quickly checked, and the head was crowning, and the contractions were now constant. I had pulled over at the right time. They were not kidding that it was time.

I said, "It's all yours," and I quickly made sure we had the neonatal equipment ready and Salt got set to deliver. The smile on her face would have been so big but she had put on a mask and I could feel the warmth from her heart. Sadly, the dad was not present, and it was not the ideal delivery location, but we would make the best of the situation. He was supposed to be following us, but we had been speeding and he would hopefully catch up to us soon.

I suddenly noticed the dad's car pulling up behind our unit, and I quickly ushered him into the unit. Salt and Pepper were in the process of getting the head out. In seconds, we had a cry, and as Salt checked the baby's neck, the umbilical cord was wrapped around it. We tried to lift it off, but it was too tight. I quickly reached in with clamps and we cut the cord. As soon as that was done, the newborn was free to come out the rest of the way. It was a little girl and she was beautiful. The crying was perfect in my world and her colour quickly changed to a nice pink. We dried her off and she was quickly placed on the mom's chest for some much-needed bonding and love. The dad was smiling, and the mom was beaming with delight. We noticed the backup unit pull up behind us. Thankfully, we hadn't needed them, but we kindly asked if they could drive so that we could continue the care on route to the delivery hospital. They could worry about the placenta delivery; it was not something we had to delay transport for, we just had to ensure that there was no heavy bleeding and then we would have a rather uneventful delivery.

The rest of the trip was uneventful with the newborn content to be held by the mom and the dad following us in his car. We wheeled the mom and the newborn up to the delivery room where the staff quickly took our report and transferred care of the family to the experts. The crew was beyond ecstatic. Of all the calls we would do, this would be one I would remember the most fondly. I looked at both Salt and Pepper and I told them, "You owe me a Timmy's for the extra stress, my friends." As we cleaned out the unit, they were so happy. It was so nice to see such keen dedication from them, making the shift so rewarding. Not everything we do has this positive of an outcome, but when it happens, there's no better feeling. Pepper elected to drive us home and I willingly sat in the back, to let them see the world from the front of the unit. They were both on cloud nine and I would not take it away from them.

After we grabbed a coffee, we headed back to base. It was time for me to think about the many deliveries I had seen, and it made me proud to know that some parts of the job could be so rewarding. I asked the two of them if there was anything they would want to do differently next time and they both thought about it for a moment. Then one of them quietly said exactly what I prayed they would say. She said, "We need to take the next NALS course," by which she meant the Neonatal Advanced Life Support course. The fact that they both demonstrated their appreciation of the complex world of maternal deliveries made me so proud. I complemented them on the job well done and how prepared they were for this delivery. For the most part, I had not needed to give any advice and I had only quickly clamped the cord and cut it, as I had seen this complication several times in the past.

Over the years, I have seen many deliveries go quickly and most occur without complications. But there have been times that we have done CPR on a newborn for over an hour with devastating outcomes. To lose a newborn is hard on everyone. We often blame ourselves, but it usually happens for inherent reasons that we could not change or control. Neonatal complications can occur due to the mom having any one of a number of common medical conditions. The most common one is diabetes, but complications can also occur due to drug use and alcohol use before or during the pregnancy. Other bad complications can occur as a result of the effects of trauma or trauma-related injuries. I have seen terrible outcomes for the baby and the mom after falls and car accidents. Then there can be placental problems, maternal hypertension and many other medical complications that increase the risk of death for both the mom and the unborn child.

Early in my career, I attended the unplanned delivery of twins after the mom did cocaine. Thankfully, I had taken the NALS course shortly before. That night was a long night for everyone. Sadly, we were only able to save one baby that long, dark night. Despite having the proper training and the right team members, the outcomes can still be less than optimal. It was after this night that I learned it was okay not to be a neonatal specialist. I realized we all have parts of our job we won't be the best at and that was okay. It was okay to know where your weaknesses lay and when to seek expert consultation early in order to make the outcomes even better.

Salt, Pepper and I continued our informal debriefing at the base, where we talked about the call and the good things that occurred, and then we all had the chance to say what else needed to be said: That we all needed to keep up on our training and seek out expert-level courses whenever possible. I called attention to the fact that they were newer staff members and had just not had that many calls under their belt. They were new professionals in the EMS world who simply needed the time to accommodate their learning and achieve the experience needed, for nothing is a better teacher than time in such a demanding profession.

The fact is that we can always take the supplementary courses that are available to us, and even though it's not mandatory do so, it is essential for us in order to do our job better. Sometimes we take a course for our own personal satisfaction or as a challenge. It's never a bad thing to seek wisdom that lies outside of one's comfort zone and to expand one's educational level. I signed up for an advanced alcohol intervention course many years ago. It was very helpful for me to understand the effects of alcohol, the needs of alcoholic patients, and how to best intervene when the common thinking is that the patient is beyond help. In the course, I learned how other professions dealt with the effects of alcohol and how we could better serve a community where alcohol abuse was all too common. It made me realize that although we learn many things in our day-to-day work, we also need to take the time and work with other professionals to understand how we can better help patients with extenuating factors. The fact that our new paramedic programs are looking to add a community component to the program gives me hope that we can also help meet the needs of people who have been out of the reach of health care professionals for far too long.

The next topic we started to discuss that night was when to seek the next level of training to become a paramedic. Some people say you need one to two years' on-the-job experience first, and some people say it depends on the student. I said that next goal for them both should be for them to become advanced care paramedic (ACPs). They both looked at me and wondered when they would take that next step. I said, "It simply demands a certain degree of maturity, but you also need to be comfortable with your BLS skills." They also needed to be more than confident in their ALS assisting skills to ensure they were ready for the next step. I said, "You should only apply if you feel ready."

By working hard and excelling at the day-to-day calls, you gain the maturity to master the harder calls that will start to show up from time to time. Being ready to become a paramedic is different for everyone but before you take on that personal challenge, you need to be mentally and physically prepared to commit to at least two years of working extra hard to become the best you can be. It's also a huge financial cost, so it's sometimes nice to have your life in order to ensure a better chance at success. I brought up the fact that if we wanted our profession to grow, we all needed to get the extra education to attain credibility. Ideally, a degree should be the minimum goal as a paramedic, with a masters' level degree for educators and doctorate level for leaders in the profession.

The days of minimal training, and "scoop and run" are all but over. The more education we can get, we will ultimately drive the advancement the profession so needs. If only I was young again and I could be in their boots, I thought, I would love to help them change the world. After seeing and listening to them both, I knew it was my time to bow out. They would take over my desire to change the world. One day in the not-so distant future, they would be years ahead of me in terms of experience. Some of the lessons I'd had to learn the hard way, they already knew. They would not need to make the same mistakes. They could bypass the weaknesses I had and shimmy up the tree of knowledge. I just knew they could be much more then I could ever be, as they had simply started with a better knowledge base. That's how progress works.

My backup on my days off.

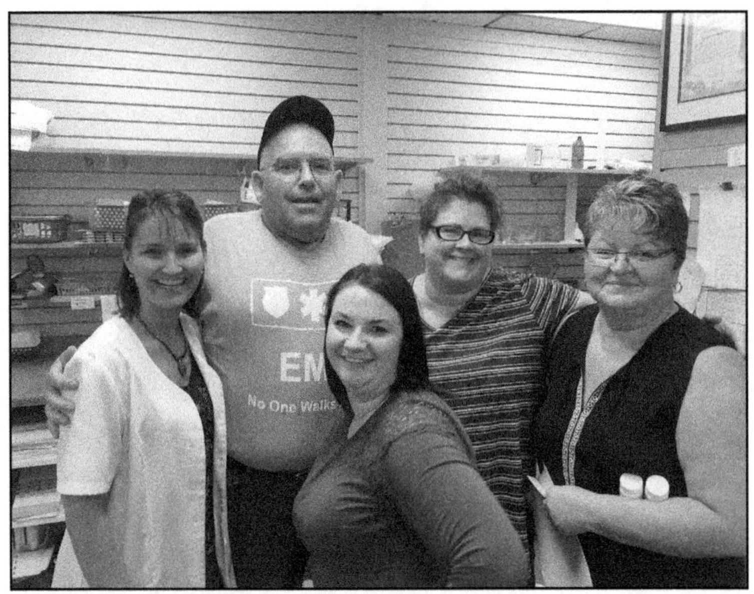

Friends will never let you down. They always know how to cheer you up.

Chapter 20: Breaking the Limits

"Making a Difference"

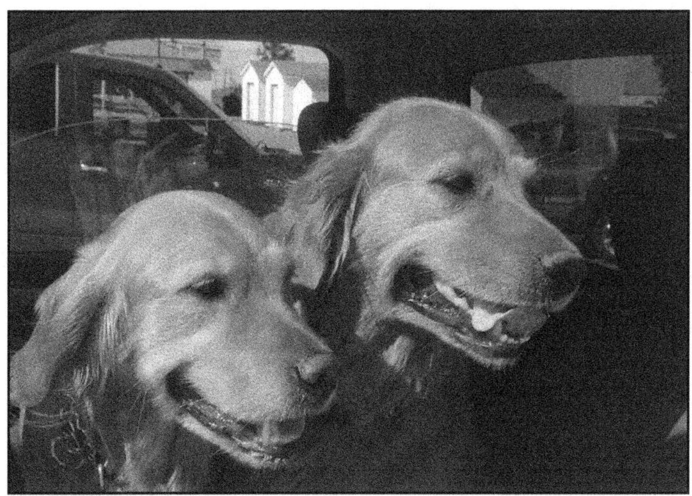

The only way to succeed in EMS is by giving 110% to everybody we touch, everything we do, and by making the best of our day of helping others in need. What we do as a paramedic or as an EMS crew is help people in need of care following a traumatic or a medical emergency. The skills we employ might be as simple as therapeutic touch, or as complex as attending to a cardiorespiratory arrest. We also provide complex medications at just the right dosage and the right concentration, and we commonly provide oxygen to patients. We stabilize patients and splint bad fractures, and for everything we do, we need the training and confidence to make the best use of our skills at the right time.

One part of the job that many people don't appreciate is that it takes much more than learning a set of skills to become a paramedic. It takes a wealth of knowledge to understand what medications will be the most effective in any given situation. The skills associated with paramedicine have evolved along with the profession. The fact that we are using more complex monitors, as well as diagnostic tools that help facilitate our investigation of our patients' conditions, is so heartening. The use of ultrasound technology, such as the FAST scan, has been a great advancement in the prehospital care profession. I would say that the skills that make a good paramedic are skills that we should not take for granted.

One thing we definitely can't take for granted is good airway skills. The fact that we can provide just the right medications, then insert a special tube to help someone breathe, is just incredible when you think about it. We have been performing the advanced skill of intubation for many years, but we also have not made the profession realize it's not as easy as it is made out to be. Anyone who has had a bad day trying to intubate someone will be the first to admit you can't just intubate everyone easily. If any one person says they are good at intubating after being supervised on only a few intubations, they truly don't get it. Sadly, many educational institutes want to churn out paramedics in the easiest and quickest fashion. There is nothing like repeated difficult or less-than-optimal situations to help a student perfect the skills needed to intubate.

One day in my last weeks of mentoring, we were called to a quad accident. It had occurred in an isolated spot and it was a longer than ideal response time. We had no air backup due to bad weather, so we had to rely on ground transport, at least until the storm cleared. My partners were Sarah and Julie. All we knew was that it was a high-speed accident at a local gravel pit. We often saw an increase in quad accidents on long weekends and in the summer months. Most of us hated working the May long weekend, as it was often the worst weekend of the year for accidents. Boating disasters and graduation parties gone wrong could easily wreck a quiet weekend.

Few things surprise me when it comes to the degree of complications that result from a quad collision. The most common effects were traumatic head injuries, chest injuries and pelvic fractures. Then came the limb injuries and lacerations. Often, there was alcohol involved, along with excessive speed as a factor, and the patients were often not wearing helmets. When you added these common factors together, you had just the right combination to kill someone. The only good outcome on many of these traumatic calls was that people on the waiting list for transplant organs got a call.

Before we arrived at the collision, we all planned ahead how best to handle the injured patient. I would do the IV, Julie would help with the monitor and then help with medications. Sarah got delegated to take the airway and I was her backup. As we approached the scene, we were met by the local police who guided us to the accident spot. We also had several volunteer firefighters arrive in their private vehicles, as they were closest to the collision scene. They had the volunteer fire truck on the road but could not easily access the gravel pit, as it was too muddy. The report we got from them was short, and it was bad. A kid with a bad head injury was the quick version. As we approached the patient, we got to see the terrible results of speed and a quad crashing onto someone's head. It was almost always a losing event.

We quickly assessed the patient and knew it was going to be a "scoop and run" call. I knew the head injury was bad from the snoring sounds that he was making trying to breathe. By the look of his head, we needed a neurosurgeon, and sooner than later would be helpful. If we could just grab him and go, do everything on the way, it would save us time. I had started IVs at one-hundred miles an hour with a two-week-old child in distress, but there needed to be a fantastic driver and good road conditions. Today, it was not going to be an easy intubation, and the road conditions would make it a rougher than normal drive, at least until we got onto the main highway. We would also have loved to intubate on route, but intubating is not an easy skill, especially while driving. I'd done it before, but the circumstances needed to be ideal. Today they were not even close to ideal. So, everything we needed to do would have to be done on scene. Then we could safely initiate the transport. Today, it would take all of us and a team effort to make a success story even a remote possibility.

It took us at least thirty minutes to stabilize the patient. The intubation was not easy, but it was done, and very skillfully done, even if we were all very nervous, for obvious reasons. When you start off with a hypoxic patient, along with a bad facial smash, it was nothing short of a miracle to get him stabilized for transport. As we loaded him up, the crew was careful to secure the scoop to the stretcher and to ensure the straps were all correctly tightened so that the patient didn't slide around on the rough roads. It may not seem like a big deal, but it is well documented that only one-third of patients had shoulder restraints on during transport. It is also notable that many staff are negligent in securing spine boards and scoops to the stretcher. This just makes sense, but it is often missed. We ensured that when we were teaching our students we reminded them to always buckle their patients in using all the straps, as well as shoulder restraint devices, so that in the case of a crash, they would not be ejected off the stretcher.

Over my career, I have seen or been involved in two separate ambulance collisions where patients had not been secured correctly. Injuries to the patient or staff can occur due to not having the patient secured to the stretcher or the spine board, but also if they are not secured correctly. I have seen attendants get hit by flying equipment in an ambulance crash, as well, and this can be just as dangerous as the initial crash. Another important step is for us to sit down and buckle up whenever possible. We must also ensure we have secured equipment prior to transport and during transport, just in case we ever had a crash or if the driver has to hit the brakes hard. The airway kit, Physio monitor, drug kits and IV pumps are all heavy and can easily fly around during transport.

The netting that is now on all units is called the "EMT catcher" for a reason. When the driver hits the brakes, the attendant flies into the netting. It has caught me more often than I want to admit. The safest seat is closer to the netting than farther away. Commonly, there are three seating positions on the side bench. Always ensure that your partners are buckled in, if possible, too.

The driver must always take extra care in driving when the crew is working on a patient in the patient compartment. My driver always knew to take it extra slow around the corners. They would often call out the road conditions or let us know of bumps or turns before they occurred. It is totally different driving with a patient than when there is no patient in the back. We would often need to stand to change IV bags or reach extra equipment, but it was always wise to get your seat belt on, as soon as possible. As long as our partner was driving safely, we were okay. You couldn't predict when other drivers would suddenly stop in front of you or cut you off at an intersection.

The final thing to never take for granted are fatigue factors. We all have our breaking point; we also know we can only be efficient for so long and then we can start making mistakes. Fatigue, as well as being pushed too hard for too long, is asking for us to make a mistake. There are many qualities that make up a good paramedic, but there always things that can work against us. Safety is one thing we can never be too careful about when it comes to looking after our own lives and those of our patients and partners.

On route to the hospital, we noticed the patient's vital signs starting to deteriorate. Julie was driving as quickly but as safely as possible. Sarah and I were busy trying to keep the vital signs within the proper range. We were giving IV boluses and positioning his head slightly higher than his body to help decrease the cerebral swelling. There was not much else we could do other than to ensure the ventilation rate was high enough to ensure the CO2 was maintained at the right range. We were diligent in ensuring the oxygenation was in the higher range to keep the brain adequately oxygenated. We consulted the OLMC and added the drug, Mannitol. Normally, we needed a CT scan done first, but things were looking bleak, it was the best course of action. If only we had an air transport, we could have cut down the transport time, but as Mother Nature had her own agenda, we made the best of the current situation.

After we started the Mannitol, the patient's condition improved; we had bought the patient some extra time. We were cheering when we heard our driver tell us we finally hit the highway and could make up some time. The last twenty minutes of rough road was not much fun for anyone. But in no time at all, we were entering the city limits, and the trauma team was ready to take over upon our arrival. Our report and transfer of care to the trauma team staff was unremarkable. Thankfully, a neurosurgeon was among the team. He was aware of the treatment and potential for a devastating head injury. As soon as the CT scan and the definitive diagnosis was made, some very quick and aggressive action would hopefully help change the outcome. After we got the patient onto the trauma table, we were free to go back to our unit and clean up the mess.

As we rolled the stretcher to the unit, I reflected on the fact that we had done everything we possibly could for the patient. I said to my crew, "We've done a very good job regardless of the outcome"; it was a good job. After we had cleaned up the unit, we had a chance to go back to check on the patient's outcome. My suspicions were confirmed, and the patient was already in the OR, having surgery for a closed head injury. He had a pelvic injury and spinal fractures, but overall the outcome was favourable. Only time would tell the real outcome. We had followed the goals of trauma care, as closely as possible. The only other thing we could have done was get a backup unit to our scene, but thinking back, it was not needed. If we'd had extra help on scene and during the transport, it wouldn't have changed the care.

One the way home, we talked and reviewed the call's events. The only thing that I could think of that would be helpful was for my co-workers to audit the ATLS course as soon as possible.

The Advanced Trauma Life Support (ATLS) course would just enhance their skills and training. Every course we take enhances our professional skills and abilities.

After taking the International Trauma Life Support (ITLS) course and the Advanced Trauma Life Support (ATLS) course, caring for trauma patients became so much easier for me, as the courses helped me become more organized and logical. Mastering the courses, you can perfect your care, and be better prepared for the situations you will be presented with throughout your career. Another course I think is very good is the Advanced Medical Life Support (AMLS) course, but they are not utilized as much as they should be.

The educational institutes do a great job, but there is only so much you can teach a student in the relatively short time frame that encompasses a course of study. There are only a few mandatory courses, and over a lifetime you can attend many other courses that make you a better practitioner. No course is a waste of time if one's mind is open and one's desire is keen to expand one's base of wisdom.

After we had returned to the base and restocked our unit, we all sat around, and everyone seemed a little too quiet. Sarah slowly made the rest of us feel better with her outlook on the events; she was always positive. We talked about our role in the call, wondering what we could have done better, even knowing we had done the best job possible given the situation we had been presented with. Then we realized that the only way to change the events we saw today was to prevent a similar collision from happening in the future. By working with the students at our local schools and by presenting them with the tragic outcomes of these calls, we could hopefully prevent at least one such call in the future.

I left it to Sarah and Julie to prepare a presentation about all the reasons not to drink and drive or drive a quad in such an unsafe manner. By visiting local high schools and different clubs in the community and by presenting our plea for change, we might save a life. That was part of the role we needed to play in the future of our EMS system. We needed to work on developing our role as patient advocates and part of that role would be to educate the public on the prevention of collisions.

Working as a team with the just the right people makes our world a better place.

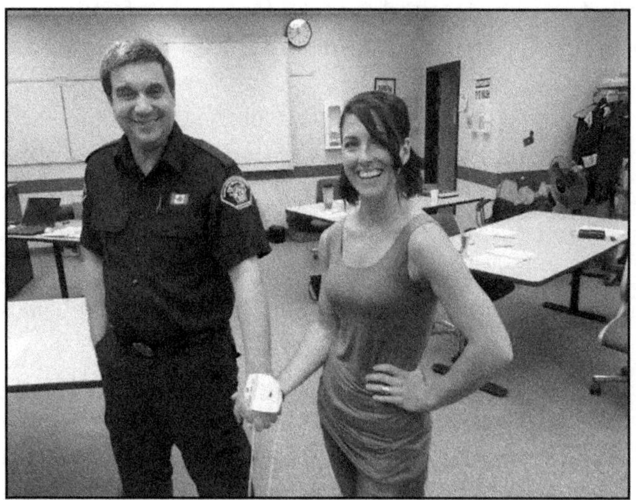

Teamwork - patient advocates 24/7

Chapter 21: Ready for Change

"Transition to Being a Better Person"

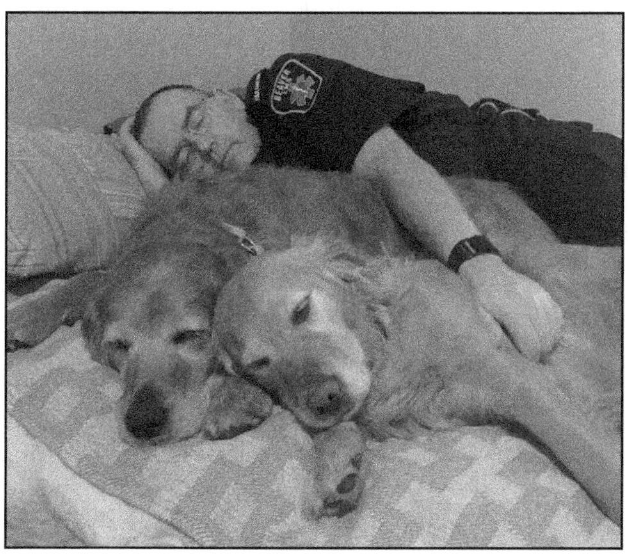

There comes a time in life when you need to start looking after yourself. You can only carry the burdens of others for so long. After a lifetime of helping others, I needed to let go of my passion, and transfer my desire to others to carry on my efforts. The time had come to walk away and let others take over my mission to heal the sick and broken people of the world. I would continue to do my part by teaching others the knowledge I had gleaned over the years, and sharing my wisdom and passion with the world.

I was so happy the day Sarah was to become a solo medic on her own unit. I had witnessed the start of her professional life and was confident she was the one person who was going to change the world. Sarah was ready to take over the unit and was the advanced life support (ALS) advocate from now on. It would be a team effort, with Julie watching her back. Julie and Sarah were perfect partners; they were like Salt and Pepper in how they complemented each other. The team was stronger with the two of them being partners. I knew that they would have fun on the job, just as they would be very supportive of each other. I was also only one call away, if they needed backup. I would be assuming the role of acting supervisor while one of our main supervisors was on holidays. Being promoted to supervisor on the PRU for my remaining time working was going to be a blast. I could pick and choose how much I wanted to be involved in the patient care, as the crews were more than comfortable to take on their roles as BLS or ALS teams. I would just be their backup and do the odd call from time to time, while other units were responding.

This particular day started out with us all doing our unit checks and we had one deep clean on the BLS unit that took us no time to get done. Salt and Pepper were the BLS crew, while Sarah and Julie were the ALS crew. The PRU was stocked with BLS, airway, ALS kits, an LP-15 monitor, extra disaster equipment and supplemental oxygen in case of an MCI. I could easily handle any emergency until the transport unit arrived. I could drive quicker to the scene as my unit had 4x4 capabilities, and I could almost float on air as long as I never stopped. Once you stop moving in water or mud, you're done. I could transport one patient on a portable stretcher if needed, but it was not ideal. The only thing I had scheduled for the day was a simple school presentation and the rest of the day would hopefully be uneventful. After the unit check and the base duties were done, we headed to Timmy's for a coffee.

While at Timmy's, we chatted about various changes in society, and how we could best help our community in light of the fentanyl crisis, the illegal drug trade and the drunk-driving rates that never seemed to decline. It was decided that elementary and high schools were the best places to start. A local school was planning ambulance tours where we would show the students through the unit in small groups. We wanted them to see the equipment, and they needed to understand the effects of drug and alcohol use. I thought that if we could reach the students on an individual basis, we might be able to help stop the downward spiral of drug use and abuse. I also brought up the fact that we needed to get an Emergency Medical Responder (EMR) program running in schools.

We had just returned to our units when we were called to a multiple vehicle collision. At the same time, we were called to a local store for an allergic reaction. I said, "You guys take the MVC and I'll take the allergic reaction. They can send a transport unit to my location and as soon as I can clear, I'll back you up, if needed." I never realized it would be them backing me up. It felt strange to watch them both hit their lights and sirens, heading south, while I had to turn on my lights and sirens to head north. I felt like I was abandoning them, but this was how it was. We needed to split our resources and make the best of the situations we were called to. Dispatch updated me of the events and that there was a transport unit coming to my location and that STARS could be launched to the MVC, if required. I would leave that judgment call up to Sarah and Julie. Salt and Pepper could handle themselves and would seek help, if they thought it was needed. So much for me taking it easy and relaxing today.

On my arrival at the local store, I parked as close to the entrance as possible, grabbed my kits and my monitor and headed inside to find the patient. I was taken to a small office and presented with a patient in acute respiratory distress. She had hives all over her body, with no adrenalin or EpiPen® available. She was about thirty-five years old and this was her second bad reaction. She gasped and told me that the last time this happened she needed intubation, which made me very nervous. I asked the radio dispatcher to speed up my backup, and asked for any additional help, if available. I would need to get to work and make the best out of the situation. I would give her every medication I had right off the start and try to abort the intubation, as it, too, had its complications, even if it could save a life.

I quickly applied the monitor and grabbed the adrenalin, and gave the EpiPen® 0.3 mg to her right lateral thigh. I applied high-flow oxygen right off the bat. I started an IV and gave the first litre of saline wide open, or as fast as it would go, as her BP was low; that meant it truly was anaphylaxis. When a patient's BP crashes, it is a form of decompensation and we all knew it as one of the true medical emergencies. I added the other rescue medications: Benadryl 50 mg IV, slow, and Zantac 50 mg IV, up and running as fast as I could get it going. I started a nebulizer of Ventolin and Atrovent, as she was showing pronounced wheezes and very hypoxic. I need all the help I could find. I inserted a second IV to be ready for other emergency medications or a vasopressor, if needed. I was about to think I was winning, when I looked at the monitor and it started to sound that there was a ventricular tachycardia (VT). I had a weak pulse and her mentation was altered, so overall, she was now unstable. I needed backup, and my backup was at their own disaster.

Looking at the patient, I wondered if the ventricular tachycardia (VT) was from the adrenalin, Ventolin or from the hypoxia. Regardless of the cause, I think I was just a little late arriving and my best option now was to try to cardiovert her, and if that failed, I would be doing CPR. I synched the machine and charged the LP-15 to 200 joules. I prayed it would help, as I wanted to first "do no harm," but at this point I was heading down a bad road and her life was in the balance. As soon as I shocked her, she came right back into a sinus tachycardia (ST) and I took a breath of fresh air when she voiced her objection at being shocked. Many years ago, an old army doctor said to me, "If you have anaphylaxis and you get ventricle tachycardia after the adrenalin, it's not a big deal, for you just caused it and you can fix it. Shock them right away and they will come back." He was 100% right. I will never feel as good as when I see someone in serious trouble suddenly turn around because of applying a quick cardioversion. It's a pure adrenalin rush for me. I was able to take a step back and reassess the situation, and the patient.

As I was reassessing the patient, who should come through the door with a stretcher but Sarah and Julie, smiling away. I was shocked, as I thought they would be busier than myself. I expected a transport crew but didn't have the time to check who my backup was or what their estimated time of arrival (ETA) was. Sarah looked at me and my patient and shook her head. She said, "I leave you for ten minutes and you try and save someone. That's our job, silly." Julie said in a pleasant voice, "Step aside, we got this one." Sarah said the collision turned out to be minor and they heard me calling for help, so they turned around as soon as they could get clear. "We may have broken the speed limit coming here, but we can deal with the cops later," Sarah said. I smiled from ear to ear and said to them both, "You can have this one and I can override your speed alerts."

The patient, on the other hand, was trying to die without our permission and went into ventricular tachycardia (VT). Thankfully, she still had a pulse, even if it wasn't very strong. It was obvious the patient wasn't aware of my golden rule: "You can't die on me." Now I got a chance to tell her, and she tried to smile despite the SOB (stress of trying to breathe). The crew quickly packaged her up and they were so happy to see I had administered every possible medication; despite having a rather irritable heart, the patient was now looking better. I talked to Sarah and suggested that if we had to administer adrenalin again, a smaller dose might suffice. Sarah said she could call OLMC and they could make that executive decision, if it was needed.

We met a police officer who had been dispatched to look after my SUV while we packaged up the patient. I gave the ALS crew a quick report and summary of my care. The police officer was great. He moved my SUV out of the way and was very helpful as he loaded my gear back into my truck, while I helped the ladies get their patient into the unit and ready for transport. The ALS crew was more than happy to assume care, and I was freed to follow them to the local ER. They patched me while in transport that the patient was looking much better, so I headed back to the base.

They met me at the base as soon as were done with the call and, in no time, we got our kits and supplies back in order. I thought about how the call progressed. It was initially super-fast-paced, but by the end, the call was a typical emergency call, where you could take your time, reassess the patient, and make decisions as a team. It was amazing how you could just go hard for several minutes and get so much accomplished when you really needed to. Many years of practice and being able to think fast paid off.

I told the ALS crew I was so busy initially that I had not been able to tell the patient everything I was doing. I had just been trying to stay ahead of her condition spiraling downward. It was one of those calls where ALS made the difference between life and death. If this had been a BLS call, they would only have been allowed to administer the EpiPen®, as well as some Ventolin and Atrovent to help the breathing and then transport. I was sure the outcome would have been less than favourable in that case.

After the unit was restocked, we took a break. I was thinking how far we had come in ALS care and treatments over the last twenty years. I shared this with my co-workers, but I also shared with them that it was past time for me to be responding to true life-and-death calls. I was more than happy to sit back and watch my co-workers assume the leading roles of the "caretakers" and the "heartbreakers." Of course, I would still gladly step in when I was needed, but I was ready to look at what I could do to fulfill other aspects of my life. I wanted to spend time reading and trying to make sense of the world around me. I was not into politics, but I could easily work to help EMS staff make changes to community practices, and to help students at the local schools become better people.

I so hoped my dream to make EMR compulsory in high schools would one day become reality, and the same went for making CPR and first aid mandatory in elementary schools. With the help of my current co-workers, we could get the schools online and take the community by surprise. We could save lives, and prevent illness and injury by changing the society of the future. There was no better way to change the world than to help our children seek the power to make the world a safer place. It would take some time for me to be okay with not working as much, but as long as I could keep busy with education and prevention, I would keep my mind occupied.

I had made my list of things that I needed to work on. The only criteria I had was that it had to be about me first, and then others; I had to make my life a priority for once. The first thing I wanted to learn, and master was the art of meditation. After reviewing a few books, I had a good idea that it was better for our overall health than most medications. The act of meditation reduces stress at multiple levels by taking away outside stimulation or stressors. Then it works to improve our ability to concentrate. It also encourages us to be more self-aware and to make better lifestyle choices. Meditation also helps people deal with stressors such as injury and diseases by causing the cardiovascular and immune system be less stressed and able to be more efficient. I figured that once I was no longer on call and able to relax, I could stop taking the medications I had been taking for the last several years to help decrease my blood pressure. If you look at the lives of shift workers, you'll see that many of us lead stressful lives. I had many miles of ocean I wanted to visit, and I had some very happy dogs that needed water to play in, so I needed to plan to live, if for no other reason than to be able to spoil them.

Everyone has a picture of the perfect place in the world. This is one of those places for me.

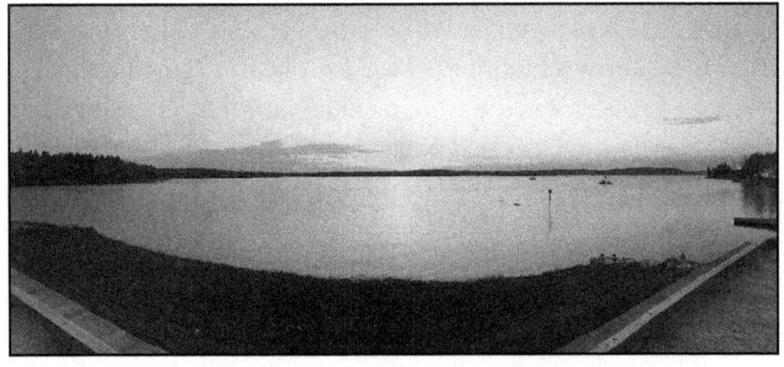

Freedom is just ahead of you if you're willing to look up!

Chapter 22: Rewards vs. Achievements

"The Ultimate Personal Satisfaction"

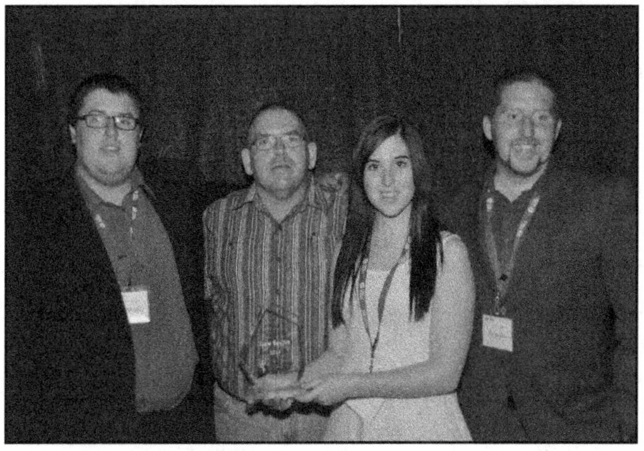

The best rewards in life are often non-monetary, and for me, in this profession, they are what we receive from our patients. To see them smile and thank us makes the job we do so worth it. After a difficult call, we are often left to wonder if we did everything we could have done for a patient. We are often torn between protocol, algorithms and actual patient-centred needs. I often look back and pray the patient did not go too long without adequate oxygenation or perfusion, and that they ultimately survived the trauma, as we often don't know the final outcome. But when you see them again a day or two later—and see that they are alive and able to smile—it is worth all the heartache and worry.

We often risk our lives to achieve this goal. Many times, we stretch our human abilities to make it possible for someone else to live.

So many times, we pick up our patients in dire circumstances and we do everything we can for them, by we never get to tell them or their family how hard we tried to help them, or how much we truly felt their pain and suffering.

You also never know just how much power your words and encouragement will have on a patient. It's very strange talking to people who are unstable and in shock, and then finding out they remember what you said, despite their blood pressure being so low at the time. We often won't even realize how involved we get in a call, until after the call is over. We form a bond with our patients from the start, especially when they are nice to us, and we go the extra mile for them.

Saving lives and helping people in need must be one of the best adrenalin rushes in the world. I may never parachute out of a perfectly good plane, but I will risk my life over and over to bring someone else out of the clutches of hell. We never seem to run out of battles with the Angel of Death, just as we never run out of good people who can use some help. I can't count the number of people who have thanked us, hugged us and cried with us at the end of a call or a transfer. It shows that even when people are at their worst, they are still so very special and so human.

Of all the interventions we perform, the one I am proudest of having mastered is the ability to start an intravenous in any position, any environment and on any age of patient. The art of starting an IV is a skill that is perfected over years of practice. No matter how many you do, you will never get them all; you will never be perfect. I think back to my last five IV starts. I had to make two attempts on two of the patients, even under ideal conditions. Attitude, along with good lighting really helps the success rate.

To be called to the hospital to help with difficult IV starts is a true testament to one's skill and being dedicated to helping others. Only once did I make it a bad day for the others around me, when the nurse I was working with got poked with my sharp. I'll never forget that day. She had to go through the Body and Fluid Exposure/Needle Stick protocol. So, even trying to help others can end up not being very helpful. We can never be too careful or too prepared when it comes to practicing our medical skills.

Another skill we can never get right 100% of the time is the simple intubation of patients. The act of "getting an airway" is not that easy. Over the years, you perfect the art of performing difficult intubations. We often attempt multiple BLS procedures, such as suctioning, artificial airway adjuncts and head positioning for airway problems. There are the odd calls where we can't get past airway and breathing assessments or interventions. Then it takes all our ALS skills and special interventions to secure an adequate airway. In the rare case, a surgical cricothyrotomy is required.

There is one skill they don't teach in school, and that is the art of holding our patients' hands: by this simple act, we are showing them that we care about them and that they have someone on their side. The act of holding a hand can do more than any medication can, in some cases. Some days, the only thing a patient needs is to feel supported or important in someone else's eyes. It's not a skill you can learn from a simulator.

Another reward we get from our profession is seeing a loved one get another chance to be with their family again. We will do everything possible to save a life. We will bend rules, speed on terrible roads, and risks our own lives, all to give someone else the chance to live another day. At the end of the day or our shift, we need to know we have made a difference to get some satisfaction from our job. After all, it's not just a job, it's a career. It's a lifestyle, as well.

Being on call, and responding to the good calls as well as the bad, is all part of our daily life. After a fatal cardiac arrest or accident, we try to see that family and friends can say goodbye to their loved one in the best atmosphere possible. This can be at their home, in the local hospital or even at the scene of the accident, which is not the best place, but it happens sometimes.

After every serious call, there is an extra adrenalin rush amongst the crew to complete the call, clean up the unit and to do the ePCR. Then we can crash. It's like running a triathlon and when it's over, you need to rest. That is the time to reflect on the call, and you need to always think about the positive events or better parts of the call first. Then you can think of the things you can improve on next time. In the moment, we must often make snap decisions, even when we aren't completely sure that they are the right ones. Making an educated guess and being right, is what we aim to do, but we all know that we can make poor decisions, as well.

We don't have CT scanners or mobile laboratories or other diagnostic tests to verify our decisions on site, but we do our best. You can't beat yourself up over the very complex calls, when you don't have all the answers; you don't know what happened before your arrival, and you are left to communicate with an unstable or unconscious patient, greatly reducing your ability to form an accurate diagnosis. We just need to do our best.

Some days we get our satisfaction from knowing we went the extra mile for the patient, even when the outcome was not ideal. We can't always win, and some days we weren't meant to in the first place. On these days, all we can do is to be our patient's advocate. By sticking up for people who can't speak for themselves, we are helping them. This is something you should count as an achievement. There are no rewards for doing it and sometimes people will not like the decisions you make, but you do what you need to do for your patients and their families.

On a bad day, when you can't seem to find the right solution to a problem, you make the best out of the situation and count that as a win. Going the extra mile for people you will never meet again is the role of a professional. If only I could go back in time and create better outcomes for some cases in which I didn't perform as best as I could, I would be able to sleep better. So often, hindsight is 20/20, though; it is all part of learning.

I sometimes look back on my career and places where I went wrong and what I did right. The fact I'm still alive despite some close encounters, I consider myself lucky. There were a few times I was in serious trouble. Running isn't usually the best option, but some days it was the only solution left. I know I stood up for many people over my career and for that I'm proud of being in the right place, at the right time, even if it cost me a few scars. Nothing in this world can pay you back for the sacrifices you make helping people in need.

Rewards vs. achievements? What is more important in this profession? I would have to say it's a combination of both.

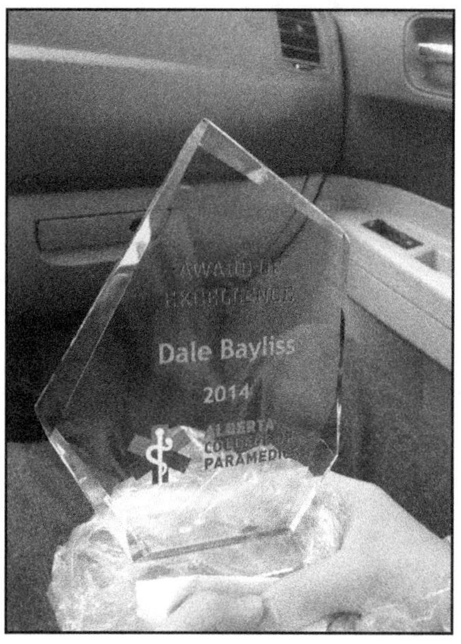

At the end of the day, I wouldn't have gotten anywhere without my friends and my EMS family at my side. They have made me the person I am today, despite my shortcomings.

At the end of the day, as you go through your career, only you will know if you made the best decisions and took the right career pathways. You are your own judge, but don't be too hard on yourself. We all make the world a better place by simply trying to do our best. That counts for much more than you ever will know. Take these words from Tim McGee from the show *NCIS* and think about your life:

"Anyone can achieve their fullest potential. Who we are might be predetermined. But the path we follow is always of our own choosing. We should never allow our fears or the expectations of others. To set the frontiers of our destiny. Your destiny can't be changed but it can be challenged.

Every man is born as many men and dies as a single one."

Chapter 23: Time to Let Go

"Walking Away Proud"

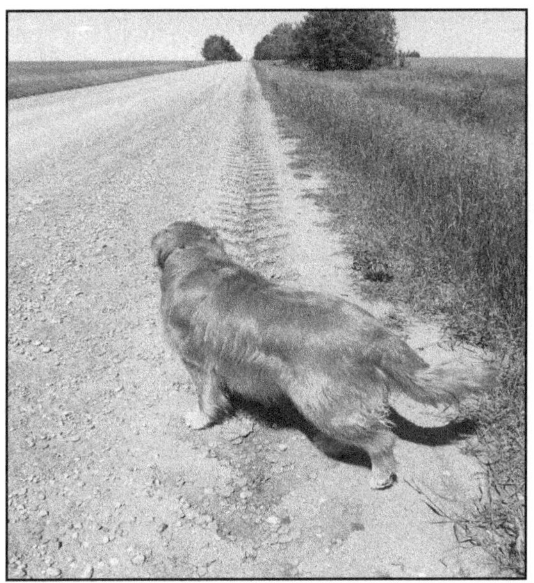

My practical career is over

The decision to walk away from working in emergency medical services was something I needed to do while still functioning at my best. Many people in my profession are very capable and they are great practitioners but being good at one's job is not the same as being the best of the best. I wanted to be one of the best, or I didn't want to be working in the profession anymore. To excel every day is what is really needed to make a difference in EMS. To only go to work for the pay would never work for me. I wanted to know that I was making a difference and that I was pulling my weight as a team member. I had a plan for when I retired: it was to continue to teach and work with people starting out in the profession, to help them be the best EMS practitioners they could be. To take a brand-new student and see them one day become a paramedic is the greatest honour. The profession could easily find someone to fill my shoes. That person will just need to know that the world is changing rapidly and that keeping up with the changes is mandatory.

Whenever I see one of my students exceeding my personal abilities, I feel humbled, but I am also reminded that I am not as young as I feel at heart. After almost forty years of shift work, your body and your mind can use a break. The ability to work, go to sleep for an hour or two, and then go back to responding to emergency calls is better left to the younger generation. The expectations are also changing. New students and staff are expected to work in a very complex computer-controlled world. Someday, we may have *Star Trek*-like equipment, and then we will be able to save even more lives with more diagnostic and treatment options available on scene.

Seeing students working as teams and learning as a group reminds us that teamwork is mandatory to succeed in this profession. Flying solo or trying to best others as an EMS student is not desired behaviour.

The ability to mentor our newest members in the profession and help them be the best they can be, only makes our EMS world stronger. We just need to ensure we have the right people coming into the profession, for the right reasons. That is one challenge that we don't have the perfect solution to, as far as I can see. There are so many variables that make a great EMS professional, but an essential trait is that we need to enjoy helping others. As an instructor, you can pick out the students who will excel from the students who won't be successful.

Seeing students take over and start to push the boundaries of our current profession is an amazing but good predictor of future leaders. The ability to take control on calls and give others accurate, logical orders is a sign that they are ready to be the new leaders of our profession. To see others with their own dreams about changing the world and helping the profession, was my ultimate dream and a lifelong goal. You can't even start to realize the pride I feel, just to know that my life has amounted to something, even if I never saw my dreams realized. I have achieved my goal of changing the lives of thousands directly and millions, indirectly. To see my students functioning as BLS and ALS providers was the best reward. The needed to let my co-workers take over and change the world. As for me, I had reached my saturation point.

For one thing, my ability to carry my end of the stretcher had become harder with the advances in technology. Our stretchers weighed more than double what we started with. If you added the patient's weight on top of that, it added up. I can remember many years ago when I started, my partner and I loaded a bariatric patient onto our narrow stretcher and had to drag her through two feet of snow for about fifty feet. It almost killed us both. Now, we would have called for backup to help us, but back then we had no backup. I remember later that night the nurses called and said the patient passed away. No matter the type of call we face, we make it work. But, in truth, it's a younger person's profession. I just didn't want to be functioning at 90% when my team needed 110% from me.

With the increased level of care needed in performing our job, I was more than happy to humbly walk away. I knew my students and co-workers could and would push our profession forward. There is no doubt in my mind that the patients of tomorrow will be looked after better and better in the days to come. Our profession is evolving. We are achieving our own independence as a professional body.

The day I knew I should walk away was when I was called to a cardiac arrest. I was driving the PRU and was just ending my shift. I was going downtown for fuel and I needed a coffee. We'd had a good tour with a variety of calls. I was the closest unit to the cardiac arrest. The police had come across an unconscious male. They put out a radio call for help. Within thirty seconds it was updated, and we were told it was a cardiac arrest. All they knew was that the patient was a younger teenager. The police officer would be doing CPR and I would back them up. Fire and our other two available units were also coming. We had Salt and Pepper on the BLS unit and Connor and Sarah as the ALS unit. Pediatric codes sucked, regardless of the situation.

As I pulled up I could see several police officers working on the child. They were in the process of doing CPR and they needed help. I quickly grabbed the ALS airway bag and the LP-15 monitor. As soon as I got to their side, they gave me a quick story. It looked to be a fentanyl overdose, but they couldn't rule out trauma as he has blood around his face. He was so small that he couldn't have been much more than fourteen years old, I thought. I passed the defibrillation pads to the member, who applied them as I got the monitor turned on. I was looking for a shockable rhythm but not expecting one. Most pediatric problems are airway or breathing-related. But with illegal drugs or trauma, nothing was for certain. The patient's heart rate was slow, and he was apneic (not breathing), which made me suspect a fentanyl overdose right away. His pupils were small and not reactive, so it was very suspicious. I grabbed the airway adjuncts and a BVM as one of the officers injected the Narcan. It was the right decision, no matter what else was going on today.

So often, we are guessing, and the differential diagnosis is not as clear as we would like it to be. There are so many potential problems and if we miss the primary problem, all our treatments can be in vain. It was then I could hear my team members coming hard and fast. Both units were making good time. The sight of them coming to my aid was so beautiful, even to me being the senior staff member on scene. I patched them a quick patient update. Sarah came back and said "Inbound angel's ETA, thirty-seconds," which made me smile. I said to the police officers that the EMS cavalry was about to give us a lesson in Lifesaving 101, and the scariest part was that they were all my past students. They all knew I would be a little on edge, as this was a pediatric code. They knew that kids were my soft spot. They could make me cry, even on a good day. I could feel Sarah's presence even before they stopped. I could hear her words as clear as I could feel her standing beside me. She simply said, "He's going to be okay," and it made me feel better as I checked the monitor one more time.

As soon as they parked their units, they swarmed us on both sides. Sarah had the crew organized and made sure everyone had a job to do. Connor took over on the chest compressions, I had the BVM in my hands and hooked up to our CO2 detector right away. Salt and Pepper were all over the IVs and, in no time, the first shot of epinephrine (adrenalin) was injected. Sarah quickly assessed the patient and let everyone know her suspicions. They were the same as those of the police and the same as mine: Query trauma, as well as a fentanyl overdose. Only time would tell if we were right, but it was a solid educated guess.

Most people think Narcan fixes everything, but if your body goes into cardiac arrest, all systems fail. Narcan can help reverse the primary effects that caused the cardiac arrest but may not fix the secondary complications. Sarah called to see if STARS was available. The signs of life were coming back. We had a weak, slow pulse and a positive SpO2, as well as an increasing CO2, which meant we were winning. Sarah passed me an endotracheal tube and I quickly inserted it. We checked the placement and were happy with it. A second IV was inserted and a complete set of vital signs were completed. Yes, we had him back. Now we needed to find his parents and get him to the closest pediatric hospital, ASAP. In a few minutes, we had an inbound helicopter with a crew that could expedite the transfer so that the critical care staff could make a definitive diagnosis.

I was slowly able to step back and watch them secure the boy to a scoop. The ABCDE approach was completed in the back of the ALS unit. The fire crews arrived, and, in no time, a landing zone was secured. The police had identified the child and his parents would be located and transported to the hospital. I said to Sarah, "This is all too familiar, my friend." Indeed, I had a feeling of déjà vu. She smiled as she looked directly into my heart. The fact that we had saved another one made us feel great, even if it would be a few days until the final outcomes would be known. We had seen our share of nightmares together.

Just before the STARS chopper landed, the boy started breathing on his own and moved his arms a little. Those were some of the best predictors of a good outcome. We had done our job. The police on scene had been the real heroes, though. The fact that they had initiated CPR had given us a life to save. A few more minutes with no circulation and no breathing, and it would have been a terminal or fatal outcome. If only we could have videotaped the whole incident and shown it to the world. We needed to educate the millions of recreational drug users that they were playing with fire. Just knowing that in our small community, one family had lost two of their three children to fentanyl made me feel sick. Thousands of people had already died already because of the synthetic homemade drug.

As the helicopter circled and made their final approach, I thought about my crews who were taking over the care of the child. Every one of them was a team player and they made the call look so easy, even if it was a complex case. There is nothing easy about saving lives. It takes a lifetime of education and a dedication to living a stressful life. But my students all knew one important thing that took me years to figure out: We are not alone in our fight to save lives. Help is always just a phone call away. I would carry my phone 24/7 for the rest of my life. They could all count on me to be their backup on their worst days. After their worst calls, I would mentor them back from hell. Even angels like Sarah could have bad days. The crews cheered as the chopper lifted off and rapidly increased its altitude. We had done it.

My career could go out on a good note. I could sign over my drugs and pass my radio on to the supervisor on the next shift, knowing the system was making a difference. As I walked out of the base for the last time, my past mentors and co-workers had my puppies and my old yellow truck sitting on the old helicopter pad. Sarah gave me one more hug and whispered in my ear, "You need to watch over me, just as I watched over you," and she cried as she held me tight. No matter what she faced I would watch over her, as my wings were paid for in blood. We would never forget the special bond we had, for it was a bond you could not break. Hell, itself had tried a few times, but we repelled the evil forces. This world would keep throwing its worst at us, but good was going to prevail. We would not lose the fight to make the world a better place. I knew it. I just knew it.

After I left the base, I went to where I normally walk my puppies. They have a pathway picked out. I just need to follow their lead and that's fine with me. The sensation of freedom was in the air, but the dread of not being able to help people in their moment of crisis was also in my heart. But you can't do the job well forever and, as we all know, there is no tomorrow for many people. I wanted that tomorrow, I wanted to enjoy watching the sun come up over the ocean and set over the land with the water in the background.

I wanted to see the whales dance and see the icebergs come into Pouch Cove, Newfoundland. These were just two of the items on my bucket list. I wanted to teach my dogs to swim in the ocean and hear the tranquility of the waves lapping on the shore. That was freedom to me. I'd take what I could today. It was time to go home and sleep with Pebbles and Ember, who would watch over me and keep me safe. Just as I would keep Sarah safe until the end of time.

Robyn and Tinsel – Tinsel's hugs were never long enough.

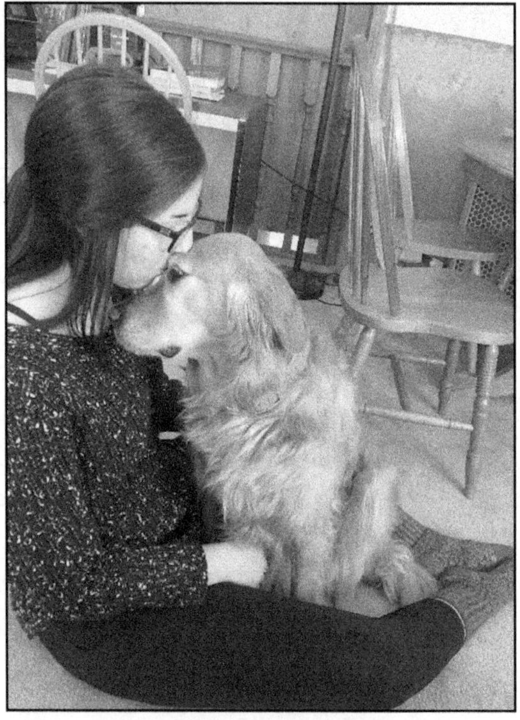

Love never lets you down. Even if it's only a memory.

Chapter 24: Conclusion

"One Last Fight against the Angel of Death"

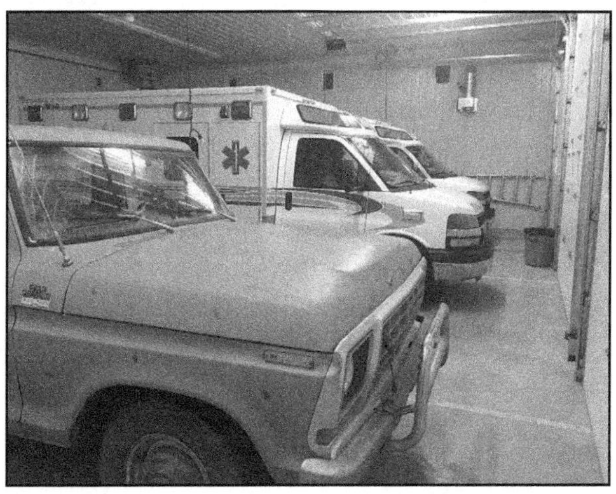

Throughout life, we come across some much bigger hurdles then we could ever imagine, but we somehow make it over them. It's all part of living. The thing to know is that we need to make it over each hurdle, or through each challenge, with the least physical, mental and emotional scars possible. Often, you can find that that you're falling before you even realize you are in trouble. That's one of the lifelong lessons we need to learn and learning it the hard way makes us never forget it. Seeing other people after they get hurt or when they are at their worst or sick is our specialty as EMS providers.

Surviving tragedies and helping others through life's tragedies is what we do best as emergency medical services professionals.

We take our job very seriously. But as we care for others, we can also get hurt mentally and physically, and it can take a toll on our emotional stability. We can be affected by compassion fatigue and post-traumatic stress syndrome, which most people know as PTSD. No one person is immune to its effects. In 2017, we lost 56 EMS staff to PTSD and its side effects. Somehow, we need to break down the barriers to seeking help. We need to educate staff, first responders and employers we can't always just suck it up and take the pain.

Throughout my life I've obtained some major scars that are visible, but most are on the inside. Only a few people close to me will ever truly know the worst moments of my life. As Kid Rock sings in "Only God Knows Why," "Every man bleeds' just like me." This is very relevant to the EMS profession. Everyone in our industry who work as a first responder has their own reasons for choosing their profession—be that a firefighter, a police officer or a paramedic—and that is sometimes very sacred. Sometimes bleeding is therapeutic, as it tells us we are still alive. The pain that is left in our big, caring and emotional hearts after a bad day, proves that just as well.

Some days we lie bleeding, broken, and hurt on the pavement, but we are not done. We get back up. If not, our friends, our co-workers and the people around us help us get back up. No matter the pathways we travel, we will cross the paths of many others who will significantly enhance and help us build our careers. It's up to us to take account of the lessons learned and keep moving forward. When we do our best, we can make the impossible happen. If we get knocked down after a bad call or we stumble in life, it's all just part of the profession we are so addicted to; it's part of the cost, and we must bear it to evolve into better people. We must try to change the world, and if only one person is saved, it's still a life saved.

When we are challenged by life's interruptions, we are forced to reassess our situations, consider our options, and find an acceptable solution to get over the hurdles we are dealt. As our career evolves, the odd roadblocks we face will challenge our own existence—challenge our physical and mental capacity—but we can make it past them with the right mindset. As we overcome life's personal challenges, we adapt, we change who we are, and we learn important lessons as well. With our will to survive and willingness to help others, we make it possible. To do our best or be successful, we need to work as a team to overcome the biggest obstacles that life can dish out to our patients and to the communities we serve.

When we are at our worst or lowest in our careers, our real-life guardian angels appear, and they pick us back up. Our friends and co-workers will come to our aid and get us up and going after we deal with the repeated tragedies from day to day. Never forget when you are at your worst that you always have someone standing over you, protecting you from harm, if you let them. You may never even see them, but they are always at your side. You are never alone. Sometimes we forget about the important people around us as we are so busy hanging on to our sanity, but trust me, they need us just as much as we need them. Once you become an EMS family member, your family is for life.

We need to count our wins and let our losses be the least of our day's work.

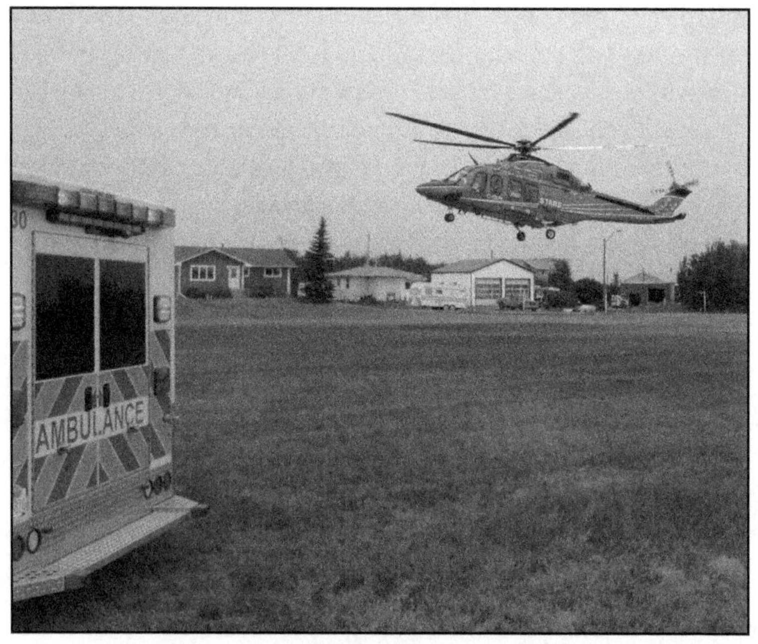

Police + Fire + EMS + First Responders = A Team of One

Advanced Life Support (ALS)

Glossary

Compiled from many current electronic sources and blended for information purposes only to clarify common terms from the MERCK Manual, Wikipedia, the ACP website, Medscape and Medline.

Adrenalin - A hormone, neurotransmitter and medication. Also known as *epinephrine,* it is produced by both the adrenal glands and certain neurons. It plays an important role in the fight-or-flight response by increasing blood flow to muscles, cardiac output, pupil dilation, and blood sugar levels. It does this by binding to alpha and beta receptors.

Advocate(s) - One who publicly supports a particular cause. We all have a passion or a cause that we care about. Being an advocate for that cause is always the right thing to do. Make your voice heard. Help those who cannot help themselves.

Automated External Defibrillator (AED) - A portable electronic device that automatically diagnoses the life-threatening cardiac arrhythmias of ventricular fibrillation and pulseless ventricular tachycardia in a patient. It can treat them through defibrillation—the application of electrical therapy—which stops the arrhythmia, allowing the heart to re-establish an effective rhythm.

Advanced Care Paramedic (ACP) - An ALS practitioner who is qualified in additional therapeutic modalities and diagnostic assessments, enabling them to provide better patient care. The ACP performs advanced assessment skills as well as basic and advanced airway skills, such as endotracheal intubation or multiple other airway adjuncts, and has the ability to administer medications by injection, intraosseous infusion or by oral routes in order to manage various conditions of the ill or injured.

Advanced Life Support (ALS) - A set of life-saving protocols and skills that extend basic life support to further support the circulation and provide an open airway and adequate ventilation (breathing).

Amiodarone - An antiarrhythmic medication used to treat and prevent many different types of irregular heartbeats. These include ventricular tachycardia (VT), ventricular fibrillation (VF), and wide complex tachycardia, as well as atrial fibrillation and paroxysmal supraventricular tachycardia. It can be given by mouth, intravenously, or through intraosseous infusion.

Anesthesia - a state of temporary induced loss of sensation or awareness.

Anesthesiologist - A doctor who focuses on perioperative medicine and the administration of anesthesia.

Angiocath - A hollow flexible tube for insertion into a body cavity, duct, or vessel to allow the passage of fluids or distend a passageway. Its uses include the drainage of urine from the bladder through the urethra or insertion through a blood vessel into the heart for diagnostic purposes.

Arterial Blood Gas (ABG) - A blood test that measures the amount of certain gases (such as oxygen and carbon dioxide) dissolved in arterial blood.

Asystole - The absence of ventricular contractions lasting longer than the minimum required to sustain life (about two seconds for a human).

Audible Crackles - The clicking, rattling or crackling noises that may be made by one or both lungs of a person with a respiratory disease during inhalation. They are often only heard with a stethoscope (on auscultation), but sometimes can be heard without a stethoscope.

Auscultate - To listen, for diagnostic purposes, to the sounds made by the internal organs of the body.

Battle's Sign - Also known as *mastoid ecchymosis*, this is an indication of a fracture of the middle cranial fossa of the skull and may suggest underlying brain trauma. Battles' Sign consists of bruising over the mastoid process, a result of extravasation of blood along the path of the posterior auricular artery.

Blood Pressure (BP) - The pressure of circulating blood on the walls of blood vessels. When used without further specification, blood pressure usually refers to the pressure in large arteries of the systemic circulation. Blood pressure is usually expressed in terms of the systolic pressure (maximum during one heartbeat) over diastolic pressure (minimum in between two heartbeats) and is measured in millimetres of mercury (mmHg), above the surrounding atmospheric pressure (considered to be zero for convenience).

Basic Life Support (BLS) - The level of medical care which is used for victims of life-threatening illnesses or injuries until they can be given full medical care at a hospital. It can be provided by trained medical personnel—including emergency medical technicians and paramedics—and by qualified bystanders.

Beats per Minute (Bpm) - Cardiac pacing, or the unit of measure for the frequency of heart depolarizations or contractions each minute or pulse rate.

Cardiac Arrest - The sudden stop in effective blood flow due to the failure of the heart to contract effectively. Symptoms include loss of consciousness and abnormal or absent breathing. Some people may have chest pain, shortness of breath, or nausea before this occurs. If not treated within minutes, death usually occurs.

Cardiac Contusion - Also known as *myocardial contusion*, this is a term for a bruise (contusion) to the heart after an injury. It is usually a consequence of blunt trauma to the anterior chest wall, and the right ventricle is thought to be most commonly affected due to its anatomic location as the most anterior surface of the heart.

Cardiac Disease (CVD) - A class of diseases that involve the heart or blood vessels. Cardiovascular disease includes coronary artery diseases (CADs), such as angina and myocardial infarction (commonly known as a heart attack). Other CVDs include stroke, heart failure, hypertensive heart disease, rheumatic heart disease, cardiomyopathy, heart arrhythmia, congenital heart disease, valvular heart disease, endocarditis, aortic aneurysms, peripheral artery disease, thromboembolic disease and venous thrombosis.

Cardiac Care Unit (CCU) - A specialized hospital unit that is equipped to treat and monitor patients with serious heart conditions.

Cerebral Perfusion (CPP) - The pressure gradient between the systemic blood pressure and the pressure in the cranial compartment. The pressure difference is the gradient that is necessary to drive blood from the aorta into the cranial compartment. Blood flow and perfusion to the brain depend upon an adequate blood pressure gradient.

Cervical Collar - Also known as a neck brace, this is a medical device used to support a person's neck. It is used by emergency personnel for patients who have had traumatic head or neck injuries and can be used to treat chronic medical conditions.

Child Abuse - The physical, sexual, or psychological mistreatment or neglect of a child or children, especially by a parent or other caregiver. It may include any act or failure to act by a parent or other caregiver that results in actual or potential harm to a child, and can occur in a child's home, or in the organizations, schools or communities the child interacts with.

Compassionate Fatigue - Also known as *secondary traumatic stress* (STS), this is a condition characterized by a gradual lessening of compassion over time. It is common among individuals who work directly with trauma victims, such as therapists (paid and unpaid), nurses, teachers, psychologists, police officers, paramedics, animal welfare workers, health unit coordinators and anyone who helps others, including family members, relatives, and other informal caregivers of patients suffering from a chronic illness.

Complication(s) - In medicine, this refers to an unanticipated problem that arises following, or as a result of, a procedure, treatment or illness. A complication is so named because it complicates the situation.

Computer Aided Dispatch (CAD) - A computer system that assists 911 operators and dispatch personnel in handling and prioritizing calls. Enhanced 911 will send the location of the call to the CAD system, which will automatically display the address of the 911 caller on a screen in front of the operator. Complaint information is then entered into the computer and is easily retrievable. The system may be linked to MDTs in patrol cars, allowing dispatchers and officers to communicate without using voice. The system may also be interfaced with NCIC, AVL, or a number of other programs

Computer Tomography (CT) - Radiography in which a three-dimensional image of a body structure is constructed by a computer from a series of cross-sectional images made along an axis.

Congestive Heart Failure (CHF) - Heart failure in which the heart is unable to maintain adequate circulation of blood in the tissues of the body or to pump out the venous blood returned to it by the venous circulation.

Consciousness - The state or quality of awareness, of being aware of an external object or something within oneself. If someone is awake, orientated and alert they have a GCS of 15/15.

Consequences - That which follows something on which it depends; that which is produced by a cause. A result of actions, especially if such a result is unwanted or unpleasant.

Cardiopulmonary Resuscitation (CPR) - An emergency procedure in which the heart and lungs are made to work by compressing the chest overlying the heart and forcing air into the lungs. CPR is used to maintain circulation when the heart has stopped pumping on its own.

Cricothyrotomy - An incision made through the skin and cricothyroid membrane to establish a patient airway during certain life-threatening situations, such as airway obstruction by a foreign body, angioedema or massive facial trauma. Cricothyrotomy is nearly always performed as a last resort in cases where endotracheal and nasotracheal intubation is impossible or contraindicated.

Critical Incident Stress Debriefing (CISD) - A specific, seven-phase, small-group, supportive crisis intervention process. It is just one of the many crisis intervention techniques which are included under the umbrella of a Critical Incident Stress Management (CISM) program. The CISD is simply a supportive, crisis-focused discussion of a traumatic event (which is frequently called a critical incident). Critical Incident Stress Debriefing was developed exclusively for small, homogeneous groups who have encountered a powerful traumatic event. It aims at reduction of distress and a restoration of group cohesion and unit performance.

Crystal Meth - A strong central nervous system (CNS) stimulant that is mainly used as a recreational drug. Methamphetamine is often used recreationally for its effects as a potent euphoriant and stimulant as well as its aphrodisiac qualities.

Decompensated Shock - This phase occurs when local tissue beds that were vasoconstricted begin to vasodilate. Vasodilation leads to pooling of blood and maldistribution of flow to non-essential organs. Clinical signs include grey mucous membranes, bradycardia, loss of vasomotor tone leading to hypotension, and severely altered mentation. The patient often is stuporous to comatose. Ventricular arrhythmias can be seen on an ECG. It is important to realize that the progression from compensated to decompensated shock can occur over minutes to hours, depending on the cause and severity of injury, and that patients can present anywhere along this spectrum.

Diaphoretic - The secretion of sweat, especially the profuse secretion associated with an elevated body temperature, physical exertion, exposure to heat, and mental or emotional stress. Sweating is centrally controlled by the sympathetic nervous system and is primarily a thermoregulatory mechanism. However, the sweat glands on the palms and soles respond to emotional stimuli and do not always participate in thermal sweating. The rate of sweating is generally not affected by water deficiency, but it may be reduced by severe dehydration; it also diminishes when salt intake exceeds salt loss.

Distention - The state of being distended, enlarged, or swollen from internal pressure. Common distention is caused by gas buildup, gastric distention or by an internal inflammatory process.

Dopamine Infusion - An organic chemical of the catecholamine and phenethylamine families that plays several important roles in the brain and body. Dopamine as a manufactured medication is most commonly used as a stimulant drug in the treatment of severe low blood pressure, slow heart rate and cardiac arrest. It is given intravenously. Since the half-life of dopamine in plasma is very short—approximately one minute in adults, two minutes in newborn infants and up to five minutes in preterm infants—it is usually given in a continuous intravenous drip rather than a single injection.

Drug-Induced Haze - An atmospheric haze and/or vagueness of mind or mental perception caused by recreational or medical drugs.

Emergency Medical Services (EMS) - A type of emergency service dedicated to providing out-of-hospital acute medical care, transport to definitive care, and other medical transport to patients with illnesses and injuries which prevent the patient from transporting themselves.

Emergency Medicine - A medical specialty concerned with the care and treatment of acutely ill or injured patients who need immediate medical attention.

EMT-A - A health care provider of emergency medical services. EMTs are clinicians trained to respond quickly to emergency situations regarding medical issues, traumatic injuries and accident scenes. EMT-As are now known as a PCPs across Canada.

End Tidal CO2 - End-tidal capnography (end-tidal CO2, PETCO2, ETCO2) refers to the graphical measurement of carbon dioxide partial pressure (mm Hg) during expiration. With continuous technological advancements, end-tidal carbon dioxide monitoring has become a key component in the advancement of patient safety.

Entonox - Also known as *nitrous oxide*, this medication is sold under the brand name Entonox. It is an inhaled gas used as a pain medication and together with other medications for anesthesia. Common uses include during childbirth, following trauma, and as part of end-of-life care. Onset of effect is typically within half a minute and lasts for about a minute.

ePCR - An electronic method of patient-care reporting used by emergency personnel to report what care was being done each time the EMS is dispatched for any type of response. Provides call details, basic patient information, history and assessment to interventions.

Epinephrine - A hormone produced by the adrenal medulla, also called *adrenalin*. Its function is to aid in the regulation of the sympathetic branch of the autonomic nervous system. At times when a person is highly stimulated (e.g. by fear, anger or a challenging situation) extra amounts of epinephrine are released into the bloodstream, preparing the body for energetic action. Epinephrine is a powerful vasopressor that increases blood pressure and increases the heart rate and cardiac output. It also increases glycogenolysis and the release of glucose from the liver, so that a person has a sudden increased feeling of muscular strength and aggressiveness.

Extubate - The removal of a previously inserted tube, such as an endotracheal tube, catheter, drain, or feeding tube, from an organ, orifice, or other body structure.

FAST Scan - The Focused Assessment with Sonography for Trauma (FAST) scan is a point-of-care ultrasound examination performed at the time of presentation of a trauma patient. It is invariably performed by a clinician, who should be formally trained, and is considered as an extension of the trauma clinical assessment process, to aid rapid decision-making.

Fentanyl - A potent, synthetic opioid pain medication with a rapid onset and short duration of action. It is a potent agonist of μ-opioid receptors in the brain. The legal form is a very good analgesic when used correctly, but the illegal, synthesized form is not a pure form and has been known to be lethal in many situations.

First Responder - A person (such as a police officer or an EMT) who is among those responsible for going immediately to the scene of an accident or emergency to provide assistance.

Glasgow Coma Scale (GCS) - A neurological scale which aims to give a reliable and objective way of recording the conscious state of a person for initial as well as subsequent assessment. A patient is assessed against the criteria of the scale. The scale is composed of three tests: eye, verbal and motor responses. The three values are considered separately as well as their sum. The lowest possible GCS (the sum) is 3 (deep coma or death), while the highest is 15 (fully awake person).

GCS was initially used to assess level of consciousness after head injury, and the scale is now used by first responders, EMS, nurses and doctors as being applicable to all acute medical and trauma patients. At the hospital, it's also used in monitoring chronic patients in intensive care.

Health Professions Act (HPA) - The majority of health professions are regulated by self-governing colleges under the HPA. All regulated health professions will eventually come under the HPA. The HPA was developed to regulate health professions using a model that allows for non-exclusive, overlapping scopes of practice. No single profession has exclusive ownership of a specific skill or health service and different professions may provide the same health services.

Health Worker - Any person who is engaged in actions whose primary intent is to enhance health.

Hemoglobin (Hgb) - The red colouring matter of the red blood corpuscles; a protein-yielding heme and globin on hydrolysis. It carries oxygen from the lungs to the tissues, and carbon dioxide from the tissues to the lungs.

Hemothorax - A type of pleural effusion in which blood accumulates in the pleural cavity. This excess fluid can interfere with normal breathing by limiting the expansion of the lungs.

Hyperventilating - Also known as over-breathing, this occurs when the rate and quantity of alveolar ventilation of carbon dioxide exceeds the body's production of carbon dioxide.

Hypovolemic - A state of decreased blood volume; more specifically, a decrease in volume of blood plasma. It refers to the intravascular component of volume contraction (or loss of blood volume due to things such as bleeding or dehydration), but a decrease in blood plasma is the most essential one.

Hypoxic Heart - Hypoxia refers to a condition in which the body or a region of the body is deprived of adequate oxygen supply at the tissue level; in this case it involves the heart.

Intervention(s) - The act of intervening, interfering or interceding with the intent of modifying the outcome. In medicine, an intervention is usually undertaken to help treat or cure a condition.

Interventional Cardiac Catheter Lab - A specialized area where a cardiac catheterization (heart catheterization) procedure is performed, that is the insertion of a catheter into a chamber or vessel of the heart. This is done both for diagnostic and interventional purposes. Subsets of this technique are mainly coronary catheterization, involving the catheterization of the coronary arteries, and catheterization of cardiac chambers and valves of the cardiac system.

Interventional Radiology Procedures - Procedures whereby interventional radiologists (IRs) use their expertise in reading X-rays, ultrasound and other medical images to guide small instruments such as catheters (tubes that measure just a few millimeters in diameter) through the blood vessels or other pathways to treat disease percutaneously (through the skin). These procedures are typically much less invasive and much less costly than traditional surgery.

Intraosseous - This refers to the process of injecting directly into the marrow of a bone to provide a non-collapsible entry point into the systemic venous system. This technique is used to provide fluids and medication when intravenous access is not available or not feasible.

International Trauma Life Support (ITLS) - A global not-for-profit organization dedicated to preventing death and disability from trauma through education and emergency trauma care. ITLS courses give the student the knowledge and hands-on skills to take better care of trauma patients. ITLS stresses rapid assessment, appropriate intervention and identification of immediate life threats. The ITLS framework for rapid, appropriate and effective trauma care is a global standard that works in any situation.

Jaws of Life - Emergency rescue equipment used to open a destroyed passenger vehicle, to quickly and somewhat safely extricate the trapped occupants.

Laryngoscope - A rigid or flexible endoscope passed through the mouth and equipped with a source of light and magnification, for examining and performing local diagnostic and surgical procedures on the larynx.

Left Main Coronary Artery (LMCA) - One of the coronary arteries that arises from the aorta above the left cusp of the aortic valve and feeds blood to the left side of the heart.

Level of Consciousness (LOC) - A measurement of a person's arousability and responsiveness to stimuli from the environment.

Levophed - Also known as *norepinephrine bitartrate*, this is an adjunctive treatment in cardiac arrest and profound hypotension. Levophed functions as a peripheral vasoconstrictor (alpha-adrenergic action) and as an inotropic stimulator of the heart and dilator of coronary arteries (beta-adrenergic action).

Life-threatening - Term referring to an illness or situation where there is a strong possibility of death.

Mannitol - A naturally occurring substance that causes the body to lose water (diuresis) through osmosis. Used in emergency situations with cerebral edema under the direction of an emergency physician or a neurosurgeon.

Mean Arterial Pressure (MAP) - A term used in medicine to describe an average blood pressure in an individual. It is defined as the average arterial pressure during a single cardiac cycle. Ideally, we want a MAP greater than 65 in any patient who is unwell and in traumatic head injury patients it would be better to see the MAP over 75.

Medevac - Refers to the timely and efficient movement and on-route care provided by medical personnel to wounded being evacuated from a battlefield, to injured patients being evacuated from the scene of an accident to receiving medical facilities, or to patients at a rural hospital requiring urgent care at a better-equipped facility using medically equipped ground vehicles (ambulances) or aircraft (air ambulances).

Medical - Relating to the science of medicine, or to the treatment of illness and injuries.

Medication Administration - The applying, dispensing, or giving of drugs or medicines as prescribed by a physician.

Mental Health Act - The law which sets out when you can be admitted, detained and treated in hospital against your wishes.

Mentor - A person who enters a relationship in which a more experienced or more knowledgeable person helps to guide a less experienced or less knowledgeable person. The mentor may be older or younger than the person being mentored, but he or she must have a certain area of expertise. It is a learning and development partnership between someone with vast experience and someone who wants to learn.

Milliamperes - A unit of electric current that is one thousandth of an ampere. Ampere is the current that, if maintained in two straight parallel conductors of infinite length and of negligible circular cross-sections and placed 1 m apart in a vacuum, produces between them a force of 2 × 10-7 N/m of length.

Mindful Meditation - Mindfulness is the practice of cultivating non-judgmental awareness in day-to-day life. Meditation is a tool, a type of training to help us be more mindful during each day. Mindfulness benefits people who experience stress in their lives as well as those who don't. It enables us to live our life more fully, effectively, and peacefully. It gives us greater control of our experiences and more satisfying ways of responding to them. It helps us transcend any images of our self and our capabilities that might narrow our experience.

Narcan Kits - Narcan is a drug that can be injected to temporarily reverse an overdose of fentanyl or other opioids, allowing the patient to then get emergency medical help. Each kit contains two units of naloxone, two syringes, two alcohol swabs, two latex gloves, a one-way breathing mask and instructions.

Neglect - A form of abuse where the perpetrator is responsible for caring for someone who is unable to care for themselves but fails to do so. Neglect may include the failure to provide sufficient supervision, nourishment, or medical care, or the failure to fulfill other needs which the victim cannot provide themselves.

Neurogenic Shock - A distributive type of shock resulting in low blood pressure, occasionally accompanied by a slowed heart rate, which is attributed to the disruption of the autonomic pathways within the spinal cord. It can occur after damage to the central nervous system, such as a spinal cord injury.

Neutralize - To render (something) ineffective or harmless by applying an opposite force or effect.

Nitro Infusion - Nitroglycerin infusion is used to treat hypertension (high blood pressure) during surgery or to control congestive heart failure in patients who have had a heart attack. It may also be used to produce hypotension (low blood pressure) during surgery. Nitroglycerin infusion is sometimes used to treat angina (chest pain) in patients who have been treated with other medicines that did not work well.

NRB Face Mask (NRB) - A non-rebreather mask is a device used in medicine to assist in the delivery of oxygen therapy. An NRB requires that the patient can breathe unassisted, but unlike low-flow nasal cannula, the NRB allows for the delivery of higher concentrations of oxygen.

On-Line Medical Control - Service utilized to provide the prehospital provider medical oversight in the treatment decisions involving patient care in the prehospital setting.

Pediatric Advanced Life Support (PALS) - A video-based, instructor-led, advanced course that focuses on a systematic approach to pediatric assessment, basic life support, PALS treatment algorithms, effective resuscitation and team dynamics to improve the quality of care provided to seriously ill or injured children, resulting in improved outcomes.

Pan Scan - Whole-body CT scans can confirm immediately whether severe trauma patients have certain injuries, but these tests could miss other serious problems if performed too early. It has been found that single-pass whole-body [CT] is very effective or specific at determining where there is injured tissue but is variable in excluding injuries in patients with suspected blunt trauma.

Paramedic - An EMT-P / PCP / ACP or CCP is a health care professional, predominantly operating in the pre-hospital and out-of-hospital environment and working mainly as part of emergency medical services (EMS), such as on an ambulance.

Perfectionist - A personality trait characterized by a person's striving for flawlessness and setting high performance standards for themselves, accompanied by critical self-evaluations and concerns regarding others' evaluations. It is best conceptualized as a multidimensional characteristic, as psychologists agree that there are many positive and negative aspects.

Personal Protective Equipment (PPE) - Refers to protective clothing, helmets, goggles, or other garments or equipment designed to protect the wearer's body from injury or infection. The hazards addressed by protective equipment include physical, electrical, heat, chemicals, biohazards, and airborne particulate matter.

Pharmacology - The branch of biology concerned with the study of drug action, where a drug can be broadly defined as any man-made, natural, or endogenous (from within body) molecule which exerts a biochemical or physiological effect on the cell, tissue, organ, or organism.

Pleural Effusion - A buildup of fluid in the pleural space, an area between the layers of tissue that line the lungs and the chest cavity. This excess can impair breathing by limiting the expansion of the lungs. Various kinds of pleural effusion exist, depending on the nature of the fluid and what caused its entry into the pleural space.

Pleural Tap - A procedure which involves the removal of fluid from the area between the chest cavity and the tissue lining of the lungs.

Pneumonia - An inflammatory condition of the lung affecting primarily the microscopic air sacs known as alveoli.

Practitioner(s) - A person actively engaged in an art, discipline, or profession, especially medicine.

Preceptor - A skilled practitioner or faculty member who supervises students in a clinical setting to allow practical experience with patients.

Pressor - An anti-hypotensive agent, also known as a vasopressor agent, is any medication that tends to raise reduced blood pressure. Some anti-hypotensive drugs act as vasoconstrictors to increase total peripheral resistance, others sensitize adrenoreceptors to catecholamines-glucocorticoids, and the third class increase cardiac output-dopamine, such as dobutamine.

Primary Care Paramedic (PCPs) - The entry-level of paramedic practice in some Canadian provinces. The scope of practice of PCPs includes performing semi-automated external defibrillation, oxygen administration, and establishing an IV. It also includes cardiac monitoring (such as Lead 2 and 12 Lead interpretation), administration of symptom-relief medications for a variety of emergency medical conditions (including epinephrine, salbutamol, ipratropium bromide, aspirin, nitroglycerine, naloxone, dextrose, thiamine, glucagon, Gravol, Benadryl and nitrous oxide). In addition, some services have started carrying non-opiate medications so that primary care paramedics can treat patients who require pain management. These medications include ketorolac, acetaminophen and ibuprofen. As of 2015, PCPs can now administer Naloxone for suspected opiate overdoses, and perform trauma immobilization, including cervical immobilization, and other basic medical care. PCPs may also receive additional training to perform certain skills that are normally in the scope of practice of ACPs, such as interpretation or transmission of a 12 lead EKG. This is regulated both provincially (by statute) and locally (by the medical director), and ordinarily entails an aspect of medical oversight by a specific body or group of physicians. See https://www.collegeofparamedics.org/ for more information.

Priority One - Emergency services in various countries use systems of response codes to categorize their responses to reported events and to describe a mode of response for an emergency vehicle responding to a call. Some paramedic/EMS agencies use priority terms, which run in the opposite of code responses.

Priority 1 - Dead on Arrival Trauma/CPR
Priority 2 - Emergency
Priority 3 - Non-Emergency
Priority 4 - Situation under Control
Priority 5 - Mass Casualty

Post-Traumatic Stress Disorder (PTSD) - A disorder that develops in some people who have experienced a shocking, scary, or dangerous event. Not everyone with PTSD has been through a dangerous event. Some experiences, like the sudden, unexpected death of a loved one, can also cause PTSD. Symptoms usually begin early, within three months of the traumatic incident, but sometimes they begin years afterward. Symptoms must last more than a month and be severe enough to interfere with relationships or work to be considered PTSD.

Rapid Sequence Intubation (RSI) - A special process for endotracheal intubation that is used where the patient is at a high risk of pulmonary aspiration or impending airway compromise. It differs from other forms of general anesthesia induction in that artificial ventilation is generally not provided from the time the patient stops breathing (when drugs are given) until after intubation has been achieved.

Royal Canadian Mounted Police (RCMP) - Both a federal and a national police force of Canada. The RCMP provides law enforcement at a federal level in Canada, and on a contract basis to the three territories, eight of Canada's provinces (the RCMP does not provide provincial or municipal policing in either Ontario or Quebec), more than 150 municipalities, 600 aboriginal communities, and three international airports. http://www.rcmp.gc.ca/

Sellick's Manoeuvre - Also known as *cricoid pressure*, this is a technique used in endotracheal intubation to reduce the risk of regurgitation. The technique involves the application of pressure to the cricoid cartilage at the neck, thus occluding the esophagus which passes directly behind it. (Only to be done by specially trained providers.)

Sinus Bradycardia - A heart rhythm that originates in the sinus node with a rate less than sixty beats per minute. Common in healthy patients but not in sick patients who are hypoxic, hypovolemic or something that is causing the bradycardia.

ST Segment Monitoring - A technique useful for detecting silent ischemia. ST-segment monitoring is more accurate than patients' self-reporting of symptoms because 70% to 90% of episodes of myocardial ischemia detected with ECG are clinically silent.

Standard of Care - The watchfulness, attention, caution and prudence that a reasonable person would exercise in a particular set of circumstances.

STARS - The Shock Trauma Air Rescue Society is a dedicated flight team that provides safe, rapid, highly specialized emergency medical transport for the critically ill and injured. Currently available in Alberta, Saskatchewan, and Manitoba although the odd flight does extend into BC for the Calgary flight crews from time to time. See https://www.stars.ca/

Stroke Disease - Stroke is a disease that affects the arteries leading to and within the brain. It is the number five cause of death and a leading cause of disability in the United States. A stroke occurs when a blood vessel that carries oxygen and nutrients to the brain is either blocked by a clot or bursts (or ruptures).

Subconscious - The part of consciousness that is not currently in focal awareness.

Subcutaneous Emphysema - When gas or air is trapped in the layer under the skin. The word *subcutaneous* refers to the tissue beneath the skin, and *emphysema* refers to trapped air.

Surgery - An ancient medical specialty that uses operative manual and instrumental techniques on a patient to investigate or treat a pathological condition such as disease or injury, to help improve bodily function or appearance or to repair unwanted ruptured areas.

Surreal - Marked by the intense irrational reality of a dream; unbelievable, fantastic.

Tactical Officer - A specially trained officer who deals in complex and dangerous situations.

Technological - This can refer to the knowledge of techniques and processes or it can refer in machines which can be operated without detailed knowledge of their workings.

Therapeutic Touch - A natural healing method for relaxation and self-help. It relieves pain, stress and anxiety, and improves sleep and well-being.

Third Degree Heart Block - A disorder of the cardiac conduction system where there is no conduction through the atrioventricular node (AVN); therefore, complete dissociation of the atrial and ventricular activity exists. The ventricular escape mechanism can occur anywhere from the AVN to the bundle-branch Purkinje system.

Tragedy - An event causing great suffering, destruction and distress, such as a serious accident, crime, or natural catastrophe.

Tranexamic Acid (TXA) - A synthetic analog of the amino acid lysine. It is used to treat or prevent excessive blood loss during surgery and in various medical conditions or disorders (helping hemostasis).

Traumatic - Something that is emotionally disturbing or distressing. It is commonly used in medicine to refer to something that is broken due to excessive force; a type of injury resulting from force or from an unnatural event.

Traumatic Event - An experience that causes physical, emotional, psychological distress, or harm. It is an event that is perceived and experienced as a threat to one's safety or to the stability of one's world.

Type 2 Acute Myocardial Infarction (Type 2 MI) - The early critical stage of necrosis of heart muscle tissue caused by blockage of a coronary artery. It is characterized by elevated S-T segments in the reflecting leads and elevated levels of cardiac enzymes. Type 2 myocardial infarction mortality is more likely due to the nature of the myocardial infarction rather than comorbidities, and independent of the underlying triggering conditions that led to it.

Type 2 Atrioventricular Block (Type 2 Second-degree AV block) - Also known as *Mobitz II,* this is almost always a disease of the distal conduction system (His-Purkinje System). Mobitz II heart block is characterized on a surface ECG by intermittently non-conducted P waves not preceded by PR prolongation and not followed by PR shortening.

Unconscious - Insensible; incapable of responding to sensory stimuli and of having subjective experiences (GCS 3/15).

Ventolin - A beta-agonist bronchodilator that is administered in the form of its sulfate, as an inhalational aerosol or as a tablet to treat bronchospasm associated especially with asthma and chronic obstructive pulmonary disease.

Ventricular Fibrillation (V Fib) - An often-fatal heartbeat irregularity in which the muscle fibres of the ventricles work without coordination and cause a loss of effective pumping action of the heart.

Ventricular Tachycardia (V-tach) - A rapid heartbeat that originates in one of the lower chambers (ventricles) of the heart. To be classified as tachycardia, the heart rate is usually at least 100 beats per minute.

Gibbs' Rules vs. Dale's Rules

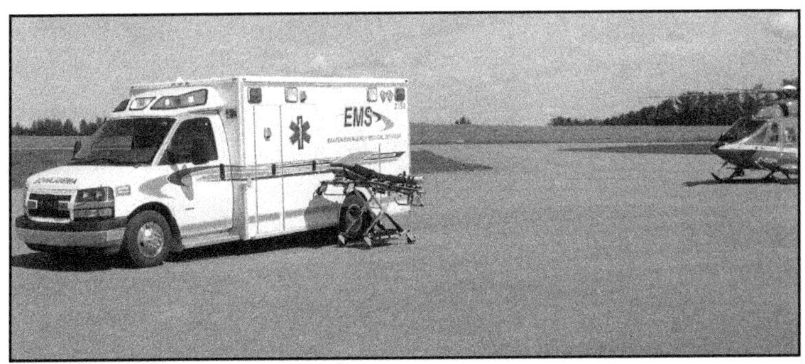

Rule #1: Never let suspects stay together. *In EMS we should only transport one patient at a time and focus on that one patient. In a disaster all rules go out the window. Also known as* **Rule #1: Never screw over your partner.** *We need to look after our partner and they need to look after us. After a call, bad things happen, so get your head out of your ass and be a team player. Don't let them fail on purpose. If you see them about to make a mistake, stop them. Talk to them. They matter, too.*

Rule #2: Always wear gloves at a crime scene. *All our patients have germs and are not as clean as you are, so wear gloves. Just remember the gloves are not that good. Just think, if our gloves were condoms there would be many more kids out there, so we need so be careful. If you get brain matter, stool or blood all over your gloves, wash it off ASAP.*

Rule #3: Don't believe what you're told. Always double-check. *Always assess your patient and don't trust another crew member, a nurse or a doctor with your career or your registration number unless you know them and trust them with your life.*

Rule #3: Never be unreachable. *Always have a backup device such as a cell phone or a VHF radio for the day your radio fails you. On your day off, ignore your cell phone and stay home—your batteries are exhausted.*

Rule #4: The best way to keep a secret? Keep it to yourself. The second best way is to tell one other person—if you must. There is no third best way. *Tell your partner your problems and trust them to do the right thing. Never lie on your PCR. If you make a mistake, tell your manager and your medical director and learn from it. Then keep going forward.*

Rule #5: You don't waste good. *Look after your patients. Sometimes you might need to deviate from protocol to do the right thing. No two cases are the same. Be ready to deviate from protocol and do what is best for the patient when the time comes. Consistently observing protocol can and will kill patients. Use your common sense and your best educated guess. You can always call a friend for advice.*

Rule #6: Never say you're sorry. It's a sign of weakness. *Never say you're sorry to the hospital staff for transporting a patient when they complain. It is their job to take care of your patients. They need to suck it up and do their job and look after them, otherwise they will find themselves unemployed in due time.*

Rule #7: Always be specific when you lie. *Sometimes others don't need to know how bad it was on a specific call, how messy someone's house was, or how someone just couldn't cope with life anymore. Some things are best kept on the PCR and not broadcast on the radio. A referral to social services, home care or to your CHAPS program can never hurt.*

Rule #8: Never take anything for granted. *If a sending hospital or physician says the patient is stable to transfer, do your own assessment. Sometimes they are just dumping their problems on you. They* *just want to be able to say, "No one dies in their hospital." You need to also be able to say, "No one dies in my ambulance."*

Rule #9: Never go anywhere without a knife. *"But in my personal life I stabbed myself gutting my friend's deer," so always carry your EMS scissors with you in a pocket. Have a spare pair for your partner as well.*

Rule #10: Never get personally involved in a case. *The best rule is never get involved in the politics of your patients' lives. Just look after the patient and care for their families. We don't need to judge their past or their present situation.*

Rule #11: When the job is done, walk away. *When the call is over, sit back or sit down and think about what you can do better next time. Not every call will go well. Some turn out very bad, no matter what. Sometimes everything goes right without your interventions. Sometimes everything goes wrong with every one of your interventions. Destiny is part of life that we can't always change, even when we want to. Sometimes we lose the battle because our patient was meant to die.*

Rule #12: Never date your co-workers. *When you work you need to respect your partner, see their strengths and know their weaknesses. Never use your position of power for favours or to get someone to do your job.*

Rule #13: Never, ever involve a lawyer. *Just do your job. There are no expectations other than to do what's right for your patient on your call.*

Rule #15: Always work as a team. *The days of the "one-man ambulance" are all but over. Funeral homes only need one person for body removal most of the time, if you can't work well with others.*

Rule #16: If someone thinks they have the upper hand, break it. *Don't back down from bad practitioners who think they are better than you. If, for example, a paramedic partner thinks he's better than you and you're an EMT, then he is out of line. If any of our colleagues think they are better than the nurses, or smarter than all of the doctors who went to school for twelve years, then they need to be medicated and sent home. Do your job. Do what's right for your patients.*

Rule #18: It's better to seek forgiveness than ask permission. *Don't be afraid to deviate from protocol to care for your patient properly. They are counting on you and patients don't follow a rule book all the time. Urban and rural EMS requirements are uniquely different. If you're five minutes or three hours away from a trauma centre with a major trauma on scene, the care requirements are going to be greatly different.*

Rule #22: Never, ever bother Gibbs in interrogation. *When you're talking to your patient, get their story. Not just the significant other's or the family's version. Patients can tell you lots just from looking at them, touching them and especially by assessing them.*

Rule #23: Never mess with a Marine's coffee . . . if you want to live. *Don't ever drive so fast or brake so hard that you spill my Timmy's. Ever.*

Rule #27: There are two ways to follow someone. First way, they never notice you. Second way, they *only* notice you. *When you drive your vehicle remember it is huge truck and doesn't stop on a dime, so drive with stopping in mind. If it took two minutes to get it to maximum speed, it will not stop fast. Just assume people will cut you off, apply their brakes in front of you, and do just about anything else stupid when you least expect it.*

Rule #35: Always watch the watchers. *If your patient is paranoid, you should be too. Never trust a crazy person. Ensure your safety and your partner's safety always. If you need backup, call for it.*

Rule #36: If you feel like you are being played, you probably are. *Sometimes you're called for the stupidest of reasons. Just do your best and take the patient to someone who cares for them. Sometimes you're doing them a huge favour just be responding, even if it is for a silly reason.*

Rule #38: Your case, your lead. *When you initiate patient care, you keep going until someone at your level or higher takes over. Never quit because you don't feel like working anymore. Sometimes you need to man up and do what's right.*

Rule #39: There is no such thing as coincidence. *Everything happens for a reason. Sometimes we are meant to lose a patient, and some calls go bad despite our efforts. Treat your patient and let destiny choose the path of least resistance. You can't defy the laws of physics with no physical or mental effort.*

Rule #40: If it seems someone is out to get you, they are. *If you have a bad partner you can't trust, get a new one, find a new job, or fix the problem. Some people are in this profession for the wrong reasons. Don't let them take you down, too. Take the high road. Do what is ultimately right for you, your patients and your service.*

Rule #42: Never accept an apology from someone who just sucker-punched you. *An idiot is the same every day. They are people who use people, discriminate against other people, and hate people in general. Have nothing to do with them. Don't give them the chance to wrong you.*

Rule #44: First things first: hide the women and children. *Sometimes we must put ourselves in harm's way to do the most good for the people who need us. Be ready to stand up for people such as kids, the elderly and the poor, who can't stand up for themselves.*

Rule #45: Clean up the mess that you make. *You make the mess, you clean it up. Sometimes after a bad call your true friends will show* *you how much they care when they help you get your unit ready for the next call. A true friend will be right beside you, making sure you are okay and that you have what you need to go on.*

Rule #45: Never leave behind loose ends. *Make sure you learn something, even if the call goes bad. Even our best effort can have devastating outcomes. Don't be afraid to go back and thank people for helping you, as well.*

Rule #51: Sometimes - you're wrong. *We all sometimes make mistakes.*

Gibbs' rules are very short and concise. My rules in EMS are very similar, but also slightly different. All in all, we don't "waste good." We help each other. Thank you, *NCIS!*

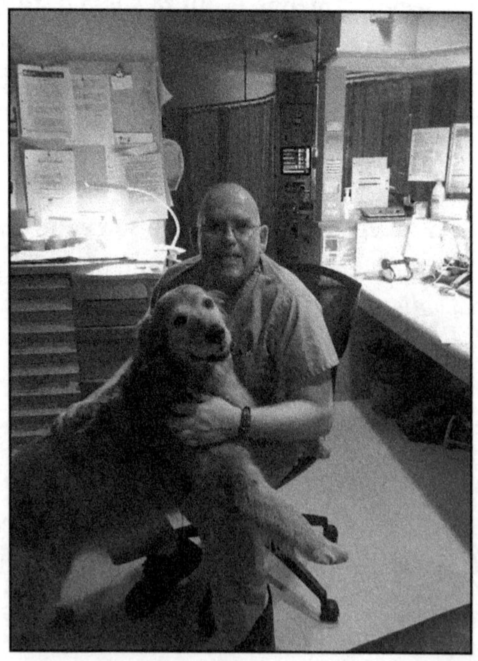

Pebbles never let me down – "Pebbles the Wolf"

Dale's Tricks of the EMS Trade / Critical Care Essentials to Know

"Eight Valuable EMS Lessons"

1. **Blood Tubing.** Using blood tubing for major trauma and GI bleeds works well. You can hang 2 x 1000 mL/cc bags and it will give the patient the minimum 20 mLs/kg bolus needed while you're initiating other methods of life-saving care.
2. **Air in IV tubing is not good**. I have a good way to prevent it. My way is a "no air" approach from the start. Always spike your IV bag upside down first with the roller clamp in the off position, and then open it while squeezing the bag still inverted until the drip chamber is one-third to half full. Then shut off the clamp. You can then invert your bag upright and open the roller clamp to the open position to flush the IV line. Then when your bag is empty, it just stops flowing and you never have to fight with air in your tubing. This is "Dale's Way."
3. **"Load and Go" saves lives.** A lesson we sometimes forget is to always assess the airway, then fix it as required or you're not done. Adequate breathing is essential, but you need to decide if anesthesia is close enough (ideally less than seven minutes away) so you can maintain an airway, then just get going. Call ahead for help on arrival. If your ABCs are stable, you're golden. Almost all basic IVs can be done on route, but you must be more than competent. Do every IV you can for your whole career and you will still not have done enough of them. You can always miss an IV, so don't ever quit practicing.

4. **Diagnosing a third-degree heart block.** When the P wave marches toward the QRS complex, walks right in and sits down uninvited, it's a complete heart block. Every one of the extra beats walk toward the QRS complex.
5. **The use of CO2 detectors saves lives.** The use of end tidal CO2 saves lives but only if we use them and correct the complications that caused the original insult. This is especially true when you're ventilating head injury patients. Always strive for a CO2 of 32 to 35 and you're good. Poor SpO2 levels even for a short time, along with or poor CO2 levels, lead to poor outcomes.
6. **Low BP is fatal.** A sudden drop in BP along with a persistent bad blood pressure and a low MAP (less than 55) equals death in trauma patients. Brain circulation must always be maintained with a MAP over 65 to have optimal outcomes.
7. **Vasopressors save lives.** Vasopressors used early in conjunction with fluid resuscitation are essential and required in many cases. Using the right vasopressor, as well as stacking or using multiple vasopressors early on, is beneficial. Most of the care we do can be measured easily enough by monitoring urine output with the Foley attached to the urinometer.
8. **Know your limitations.** Seek guidance early! When you're in over your head you need to have already called or asked for help. One example that I see over and over is EMS crews waiting until they get on scene to launch air support. Some will work on scene for ten to twenty minutes before they realize they are in trouble. By then it's too late for many medical and trauma patients. Be aware of the options as your call unfolds and seek assistance when required. Plan ahead and don't just be reactionary. Proper planning can change your patient's destiny.

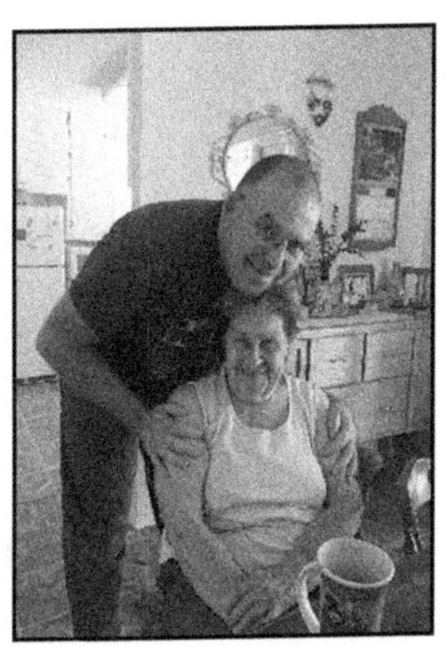

Elna - life's best educators are people we love and trust the most.

Special Dedication to Swissair Flight 111

Swissair Memorial Site – South West Dover, NB

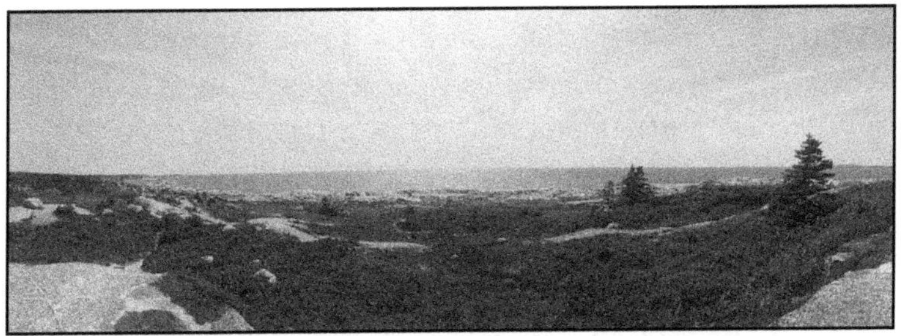

Looking directly over the crash site in Peggy's Cove. All 229 people on board perished in the disaster on September 2, 1998.

Not everything we do is about saving lives. Many times, it's about looking after the people who are left behind in the aftermath of a disaster or significant event. This picture was taken above the Swissair memorial site. It gives me a feeling of peace. After speaking with some of the search-and-rescue personnel after the Swissair 111 tragedy, I was struck with how kind people can be to others. In the face of the great loss of life, a small group of people came together and gave everything they could to support the families and the search-and-rescue personnel involved in the initial search and then helped with the recovery of the lost.

After walking the shores of the crash site and visiting the memorial, I could feel the warmth and the kindness that results from people helping people. It is humbling to know that in our busy world, there are still people who are so passionate about caring for others in times of need. The people who gave so much to help others at the time of this tragedy to know they matter to us all. They had some long and hard days. What they had to see will forever be etched in their subconscious minds.

The Swissair 111 memorial site will always be a reminder to me that despite the disasters people face, there will always be people who will drop what they are doing to ensure others are looked after despite the personal cost. I am forever grateful to the emergency services staff and the common people who came forward to give their all on that fateful day. It's a Canadian value to care for others regardless of their country of origin or their ethnic background.

We will always stand united as one.

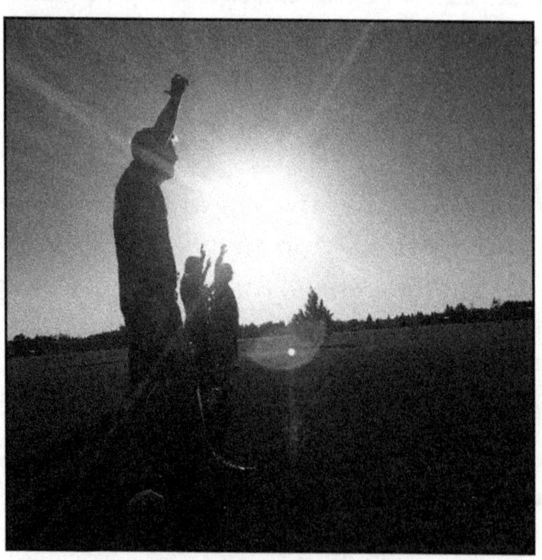

Proud to be Canadian

CPSIA information can be obtained
at www.ICGtesting.com
Printed in the USA
LVHW082229050419
613177LV00002B/4/P

9 780228 805977